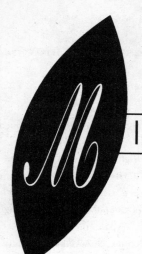

ISCONCEPTIONS

THE SOCIAL
CONSTRUCTION
OF CHOICE AND
THE NEW
REPRODUCTIVE
AND GENETIC
TECHNOLOGIES

VOLUME
TWO

EDITORS

**GWYNNE BASEN • MARGRIT EICHLER
ABBY LIPPMAN**

Publishing Editors: Elizabeth Jefferson and Sean Fordyce

Publicity: Elizabeth Jefferson

Maple Pond, Maple Ave. RR#2 Prescott, Ontario K0E 1T0 (613) 925-2111

Cover design: Beth Haliburton/Loco Design

Book Interior design: Sean Fordyce and Beth Haliburton

First Edition (Volume Two) December 1994.

Canadian Cataloguing in Publication Data:

       Misconceptions: the social construction of choice and the new reproductive and genetic technologies

Includes bibliographical references.

ISBN 0-921842-25-2 (v. 1) -

ISBN 0-921842-37-6 (v. 2)

       1. Human reproductive technology. 2. Human reproductive technology — Social aspects.

I. Basen, Gwynne. II. Eichler, Margrit. III. Lippman, Abby.

RG133.5.M48 1993   326.1'98178   C94-900017-5

Printed in Canada by Webcom Ltd., Toronto.

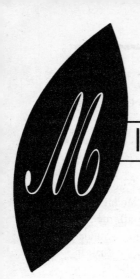

MISCONCEPTIONS

. . . .

**THE SOCIAL
CONSTRUCTION
OF CHOICE AND
THE NEW
REPRODUCTIVE
AND GENETIC
TECHNOLOGIES**

. . . .

**VOLUME
TWO**

EDITORS

**GWYNNE BASEN • MARGRIT EICHLER
ABBY LIPPMAN**

MAPLE POND, RR#2 PRESCOTT,
ONTARIO CANADA K0E 1T0

TEL: [613] 925-2111
FAX: [613] 925-0029

V O Y A G E U R   P U B L I S H I N G

ACKNOWLEDGMENTS

The editors and publishers of this book would like to acknowledge the contribution of Mount Saint Vincent University through the support afforded by the Nancy Rowell Jackman Chair in Women's Studies at the Mount to Margrit Eichler, who held the Chair in 1992-93. This allowed us to translate the French language materials into English.

Special thanks to Vanessa Hill for the very many ways in which she kept the book (and the editors) moving along; to Leopold Plotek for his support and assistance; and to friends and families who, in innumerable ways, participated in and contributed to the conception, gestation and "delivery" of this book.

CONTRIBUTORS

EDITORS
GWYNNE BASEN MARGRIT EICHLER
ABBY LIPPMAN

CONTRIBUTING AUTHORS

Rosanna Baraldi	Abby Lippman
Maria Barile	Maggie MacDonald
Gwynne Basen	Christine Massey
Ronda Bessner	Heather Menzies
Annette Burfoot	Karen Messing
Varda Burstyn	Lisa M. Mitchell
Karen Capen	Gail Ouellette
Gena Corea	Judy Rebick
Lynda Davies	Susan Sherwin
Margrit Eichler	Harriet Simand
Kate Fillion	Laura Sky
Lynn Glazier	Sunera Thobani
Sandra A. Goundry	Sari Tudiver
Donna Launslager	Louise Vandelac

Translation of Articles Received In
French by Sheila Fischman

TABLE OF CONTENTS VOLUME I

PART III: THE ROYAL COMMISSION ON NEW REPRODUCTIVE TECHNOLOGIES: A COSTLY FAILURE?

TABLE OF CONTENTS VOLUME II

PART IV: THE CONSTRUCTION OF INFERTILITY

We are all daughters although we may not all be mothers. We offer this book in the hope that it will help insure true and full procreative freedom for future generations.

PREFACE

GWYNNE BASEN
MARGRIT EICHLER
ABBY LIPPMAN

This book is one of two volumes that emerged from a collaborative effort between the editors and the individual authors. This collaboration is reflected in the alphabetical listing of the editors as well as in the generous participation of the 26 women who wrote most of the words that follow under extraordinary time and resource constraints imposed by their already overcommitted schedules. Any profits from royalties will go to the NAC Charitable and Educational Trust.

We have long been troubled by the Royal Commission and as the date for release of its report seemed to be getting closer, we felt we had to do something about our concerns: something that would open consideration of the new reproductive and genetic technologies beyond the "official" word to come from the Commission. Something that would keep the discussion open and participatory. This collection is a first step to open the issues.

The papers in this book do not speak for all women. Most important, we as editors and writers of chapters do not — and would not want to — *presume* to speak for all women.

What we offer, rather, are some voices. We asked women whose views we wanted to read and to share with others to join us. (And we apologize to those who are missing because space and time limits, theirs and ours, precluded the contributions we would have liked from them.) To the ear, some may seem political, some personal, some polemical. They are all of these, and more. They are the uneven, untranslated voices of women who represent themselves and no one else. We have encouraged this diversity, aiming not for an academic monotone but for an accessible *a capella* chorus.

Thus, the voices here speak at many levels, with many sounds. But the chorus is incomplete; many other voices need to be heard. Perhaps the sounds of concern, anger and pain expressed here will encourage the public not only to begin listening carefully to what we are told about the new reproductive and genetic technologies but also to raise their voices with us.

PART IV

THE CONSTRUCTION OF INFERTILITY

For years, feminist critics of the new reproductive technologies have challenged the headlines claiming an "epidemic" of infertility. They have shown how the spectre of increasing infertility is being used as an alibi to defend an unprecedented technological encroachment into procreation, and as a Trojan Horse, hiding the movement of genetic technologies into human creation (Vandelac).

Most often though, these serious concerns have been ignored and the feminist critique misrepresented to the public as a heartless attack on women who merely want to have their own biological children. This "angle" has repeatedly been made the major focus of media reports on the reproductive technologies. It has also become the public stance of organizations that support the proliferation of these technologies. As a result, instead of informed public discussion of the causes, treatment and prevention of infertility, public debate has been reduced to arguments for or against IVF and the women who use it. Instead of an analysis of IVF in a continuum of procreative and genetic technologies, the public is presented with attacks on feminist critics who are accused of denying reproductive choice to women.

There are no reliable statistics on the prevalence of infertility in Canada. But numbers ranging from one in six to as high as one in three couples "affected" by infertility are consistently touted by those who have a vested interest in manufacturing an "epidemic."

It is in the obvious interests of the reproductive industry to sell infertility as a growing individual problem demanding a strictly medical-technological solution. Challenging that formulation, Karen Messing and Gail Ouellette propose that infertility be viewed as a public health problem, forcing government and industry to act in ways that would protect and support reproductive health. In her piece linking infertility with childhood sexual abuse, Lynda Davies shows how a focus on medical, technological solutions to infertility diverts attention from the roots of the problem.

In her article, Kate Fillion introduces us to some of those people who undergo long, painful procedures in their efforts to have a biological child. She tells the stories of the women and men whose pictures don't appear in the newspapers holding smiling infants, the 90 percent who go through years of IVF without a healthy baby to take home at the end.

Almost completely absent from the public discussion is the recognition that infertility can be, and is, created by the same people who then turn around and offer us "cures." Harriet Simand describes the tragic legacy of DES. Children born to women given DES by their doctors and who appeared completely healthy at birth, find themselves, twenty years later, having significantly increased rates of cancer and fertility problems. Harriet Simand calls it "one of modern medicine's biggest blunders." But as Rosanna Baraldi documents, the lesson has not been learned. The Canadian Government still has no procedures for properly evaluating the long-term effects of pharmaceutical products and the potential consequences of this governmental neglect may be disastrous for women prescribed massive amounts of "fertility" drugs, and for any children they may have.

Infertility was constructed in many forms and fashions during the public hearings organized by the Royal Commission on The New Reproductive Technologies. Maggie MacDonald examines the metaphors for procreation and infertility that appeared in the briefs presented to the Commission and their implications for women and society.

Heather Menzies places the reproductive technologies inside her own construction of technology and women. She suggests, rather optimistically, that women can control the "IVF experiment" on their own terms. This is not a position shared by the editors of this book, but we include it as part of our commitment to the "open inclusive discussion" Heather Menzies calls for.

16

THE SOCIAL CONSTRUCTION OF REPRODUCTIVE TECHNOLOGIES AND OF CHOICE

Heather Menzies

When I first wrote about *in vitro* fertilization, in 1987[1], I repudiated the new reproductive technologies (NRTs) with all the vehemence with which I had turned my back on them as a solution to my newly diagnosed infertility two years previously.

I haven't regretted my choice. But I've since come 'round a bit. I've recognized that my initial outright rejection of technology as a solution to my problem had a lot to do with denial of my problem in the first place. Now I realize that I would have thought it through differently. I would have begun by acknowledging that technology permeates the landscape of my life, and I negotiate participation in it almost daily. Technology determines and shapes many of my choices, and yet it's also a social construction. By understanding some of the elements which determine its construction, I can gain some control. Perhaps I can redesign it, or redirect its application and use. At the least, I might better understand why saying NO! is truly the only choice available.

What I offer here is a reflection on the social construction of reproductive technologies and of women's choices around them. It's a reflection drawn from women's experience and use of these and other technologies — i.e. women's actual and historical technological practice. It's also an attempt to break the dichotomy which positions us either outside the technology with no opportunity to control it, or totally within its control, little more than its helpless victims.

Conventional wisdom — associated with dictionary definitions, educational curricula and media coverage of technology — reinforces women's sense of being either outside technology or on the passive receiving end of it. We are schooled to think of technology as industrial tools, machines and systems: factory production systems primarily, but also military systems and energy systems. In other words, big stuff, capital-intensive stuff, designed by engineers.[2] However, this is a restricted definition of technology, associated with capitalist, industrial, patriarchal society, which admittedly has a near-monopoly on thinking and doing around the world. However, if we dare think for ourselves and be broadly inclusive, technology can be better defined as plain, everyday know-how (Macdonald, 1987) and as practice (Franklin, 1990). At its simplest, technology involves how we go about the business of life. Not so much as individuals in isolation from each other, but as groups and communities. Commonly practiced "ways of doing something" (Kenneth Boulding in Franklin, 1990) constitute our technology. They include techniques for toilet training toddlers, tracking computer viruses or getting black currant jelly to set. They can be cultural practices — such as quilting bees, coffee klatches and consciousness-raising groups. They can be production practices — such as the crafts of cheese and cloth making associated with women's pre-industrial work; and the ongoing techniques women use to preserve food among Canada's First Nations communities and country women of Africa, Asia and Latin America. They can be formalized as rituals, such as saying grace before meals or prayers at bedtime. They can also be formalized as concrete systems — transportation systems, office communication systems, medical systems.

Technology varies from society to society and even among groups within society and in different settings — such as women in the home or native people living on the land. The key is the social relations and organization, and the values inspiring them. Because what emerges as the customary way of doing things and how this is formalized as customs and systems depends on the prevailing world view, including what is seen as valuable and important to the people of that society or group. A society which values power in the form of control might privilege tools of combat and competitive ranking systems, while a society valuing personal power might privilege tools of creative self-expression, and cooperative associations. Gardeners in a community might value the personal relationships associated with membership in a local horticultural society. So, they might share their gardening technology (seeds, tools, techniques) freely. However, a seed or gardening company would likely regard its know-how as proprietary, and seek both to patent what seeds and techniques it can and to sell others through gardening services.

The corporate, competitive, controlling perspective is the dominant way of seeing things in our society. It has been called the "dominator model" (Eisler, 1988) and is represented both as patriarchy and in capitalism, where the ability to amass money (through the production and marketing of goods and services) is the medium of control. There is a dominant technological practice associated with this world view. My friend Ursula Franklin calls it "the production model"(Franklin, 1990). It's a top-down systems approach, through which everything from the identification of problems and needs to the articulation of solutions — in the form of commodified goods and services — and the production and delivery of those solutions, through instructions, prescriptions, protocols and practices, is controlled through designated ranks of people. Although the production model is best known in factories and offices, it has spread into health care and other social services as well. Sometimes described as the "medical model," it helps explain why one response to problems such as infertility and breast cancer is favoured over others — namely, individualized, commodified treatments versus collective, social and environmental measures for healing and prevention. However, this production-model practice will only become the exclusive practice if other ways of seeing things, from which other conceptions of technology can emerge, are completely eclipsed from the public imagination. Hence the importance of women re-membering[3] ourselves within our rich legacy of technology use and personal practice and using it to define our own approach to technology in reproduction.

Re-focusing on women as technological practitioners will give us a place to stand on the new reproductive technologies beyond the narrow dichotomy of being for or against the mainstream production-model idea of it. Standing inside a woman-defined approach to technological practice will help us resist the production-model approach to women's reproductive health and replace it with a model of our own. For instance, the goal of assisting and protecting women's capacity to have healthy babies with a minimum of intervention and related dependency might emerge from a woman-centred analysis of women's reproductive health needs, and a related definition of technology as social practice and know-how. This in turn would give us a positive framework in which to critique others' stated goals. For example, half the fertility programs surveyed by the Royal Commission on the New Reproductive Technologies define success as "achieving a pregnancy" (Stephens and McLean, 1993), with a live birth given as a distant second way of defining success; yet the latter is what matters to most women-patients.

Such a goal would also allow us to focus on preventing infertility over time, but without excluding the immediate, and hopefully only short-term, needs of women with blocked fallopian tubes who could benefit from *in vitro* fertilization(IVF). The larger framework would help us to support these women in their efforts to use IVF on their own terms: refusing the all-or-nothing choice which many doctors try to impose — that is, consent to total intervention including a complete drug "work-up" — and instead choosing, as at least one woman I interviewed did, to do IVF without the hormonal drugs. This puts the onus on the medical-technical staff to refine the technique of removing egg follicles from women's ovaries in a normal, natural state, instead of putting the onus on women to make this work easier by stimulating the ovaries and their follicle production. With adequate support for the women-patients, the IVF experiment could be an opportunity for women to assert their power as users and practitioners of technology and to resist the production model's efforts to reduce women to objects and victims of a male and corporate-controlled technology.

Exploring this option for women would help us to open up the choices for infertile and, in the case of artificial insemination, lesbian and single women who want to bear a child. We could widen the choice from the current one of either using artificial insemination (AI) and IVF on the production-model terms provided, or not using them at all. The first option, using the technology on the terms dictated by the doctors, leaves women vulnerable to being hurt and abused. The second choice, namely repudiating the technological option altogether, leaves those women who want to bear a child, but who can't do it without technological assistance, with no hope and little support in a painful personal situation. Furthermore, both choices leave control over these and other medical technologies largely with the people who control them at present (Benston, 1993), and leave unexamined the assumption that women can never negotiate effective control themselves.

One of the first steps in developing a woman-centred critical analysis of the new reproductive technologies, from which also to explore options for women controlling some of the new technologies, is to critically examine some of the assumptions around technology itself. One is that technology is a neutral tool. A second, almost contradictory assumption, is that much of the technology operating in our present technological society is deterministic; that it is inherently controlling or inherently de-skilling, and that it exerts these biases — systemic biases, really — with an ineluctable force of its own. The third assumption is that the mainstream public discussion about technology is democratic and objective.

TECHNOLOGY AS TOOL AND SYSTEM

Popular wisdom tells us that technology is a tool, a neutral means to an end. It only takes on a bias when it is applied and used in certain ways by whoever uses it. Hence, a rolling pin or hammer can be productively used to make pastry or build a house, but they can also be used as weapons. However, the choices around what technology is developed, what form it takes and how it is marketed and represented are not neutral. These are highly political choices.

Birth control technology was sold to women as a tool. Epitomized by the pill, birth control was seen as the key to women's sexual liberation. The pill's packaging reinforced this: a self-contained circular dispenser with a clear plastic cover, it invited women to see the pill as something which did all the thinking for them, and contained its action neatly within the circumference of women's reproductive organs. All we needed to do was to take the little pill every morning. Like the IUD, the pill did its work silently. Out of sight, out of mind. Nearly 20 years later, a 1985 federal report on oral contraceptives warned that women on the pill face two to four times the risk of developing deep venous thrombosis (blood clots, which are linked to strokes) and pulmonary embolism (Rauhala, 1987).

Analyzed in the context of women's historical oppression in a patriarchal society, the pill can be seen as part of the same pattern which caused the IUD and, earlier, the diaphragm, to be developed as contraceptives. These "tools" emerged from a sexist choice that the innermost part of a woman's body should necessarily (rather than a man's body) be the site of contraceptive intervention, and that women should bear the cost and any risks associated with their use. Percy Skuy, president of Ortho Pharmaceutical, insisted that there was no bias behind the lack of male contraceptives. It's simply that the male reproductive system is more difficult to circumvent effectively without side effects, he told a reporter in 1987 (Rauhala, 1987). Yet women's reproductive systems are infinitely more complex than men's. And, regarding effects minimized by the label "side" effects, in 1985 an Ontario woman successfully sued Ortho for $600,000 in damages after suffering a stroke at age 22 after taking Ortho's brand of the pill. Ortho appealed the decision, but it was upheld (Rauhala, 1987).

The pill also emerged from a male-oriented understanding of sexual relations between men and women: namely that women's "liberation" meant that women were available to men without risk of paternity, and that intercourse was the essence of sex. I can remember the fumbled conversation mid-way into heavy necking. He: "Are you on the pill?" Me (despite awful headaches and crippling period pain) "Yes." And that was it. Being on the pill meant you were open for business. Ready, as they say, to go all the way. His way. Women are only now talking about our own sexual desires from which to begin redefining sexual pleasure.

There are important lessons here which we can apply to our thinking about *in vitro* fertilization, genetic screening and other new reproductive technologies which are being presented to women as tools of liberation and choice. For instance, is *in vitro* fertilization, which represents a major and risky intervention into women's bodies and hormonal systems, justifiable as a way to circumvent low male sperm count when sperm banks can match donor sperm according to hair and eye colour, height and weight? Is genetic parenthood, on both sides, essential or equally important, to having and rearing a child? Are there not gender differences here as with definitions of what really matters in sexual intimacy? Are we free to define what bearing a child and being a mother mean for us, on our own terms, and are we free to defend our own meanings?

In terms of the particular technology chosen for development, we could ask, if genetic screening is a neutral research tool, what priorities have pushed this technology to the forefront of reproductive health care so fast, and during a time of health-budget restraints and cutbacks? Whose goals do these technologies serve — parents who are prepared to love a baby unconditionally, or corporations and the state who want resilient workers and healthy taxpayers? And once it is in place so that this is what is being "offered" to women, is our choice and consent truly of our own making, or assumed like our compliance in "liberated" sex?

The notion of technology being in place brings us to consider technology as system. This is where a certain framing of the technological "problem" or issue, as well as the choice, use and organization of technological solutions become fixed as social practice and/or system — here, the health-care system. In both cases, the production model and related dominator mind set give the choice and organization of technology almost a deterministic bias. Time and again, preventable social and environmental problems are individualized and their resolution transformed into privatized, commodified and often ongoing treatments. The medical model, like the production model, is systemically biased toward the production of market needs, for which saleable solutions will be designed and produced by the pharmaceutical, medical equipment and health-care service industries. There seems to be no choice of technological path; the medical model one seems pre-ordained.

In fact, choices are being made. They're being made by global pharmaceutical, medical-equipment and other institutions who then market (or offer) these choices to the general public as if the consumers or users were the ones making the choice.

What happened to the Women's Health Trial for breast cancer prevention in the U.S. is an excellent case in point. Initiated in 1983 when it was approved by the National Cancer Institute, it was a large-scale long-term study to test the hypothesis that a low-fat diet could help prevent breast cancer. First, some faulty research discrediting the link between diet fat and cancer was used to postpone this study.[4] Then, the institute jumped on the bandwagon of "chemo-prevention" by sponsoring a $70 million study which involves giving healthy women regular doses of the drug tamoxifen, which is used to treat malignancies (Rennie, 1993). A similar production-model pharmacological fix, which was publicized in a keynote address at a major 1992 cancer conference (interestingly, co-sponsored by the Harvard School of Public Health and the General Motors Cancer Research Foundation), involves treating women with a patented hormone-replacement therapy costing $350 a month (Rennie, 1993).

What's happening *vis à vis* women and breast cancer gives us some important questions to raise about women and infertility. For example, where are the measures for preventing infertility by criminalizing toxic work environments, eradicating sexually transmitted disease and ensuring safe contraceptive technologies? Why has there been virtually no action toward a universal childcare system in Canada, which would allow people to combine child rearing and career development and could mitigate infertility caused by age; yet 13 hospital-based IVF and related programs have been set up across the country at a time of hospital and health-budget cutbacks (Stephens and McLean, 1993).

A woman-centred goal of ensuring and protecting women's capacity to have healthy babies with a minimum of intervention and dependency would compel us to challenge the lack of prevention as biased against women's reproductive health, and to insist that prevention be considered a top priority. At the same time, it would compel us to support those women who are incurably infertile and want to experiment with IVF. One of the ways we can support these women is by helping them critique the IVF and other technologies as given.

The key question for us to ask in such a critique is how the technologies of IVF, or AI, are organized: in an open, democratic way so that every person using the technology is able to control how, and how much, she uses it? Or is it a closed system, with little or no leeway for personal discretion and innovation by individual users? Is the technology organized so that users can adjust the tools and techniques to serve their particular needs and goals — for example, AI using donor sperm, with no fertility drug work-up for the woman? Or does it force the users to adjust to the technology, organized as a centrally controlled master plan of prescriptive technical processes and protocols — in other words, Ursula Franklin's "production model?" Built into the way technology is organized everywhere, from factories and banks to hospitals and government service agencies, the production model constantly dis-empowers and de-skills all but the designated experts at the centre, by denying the legitimacy of others' power, skill and knowledge, and by denying all but a select few the authority to demonstrate their power and creativity by controlling the technology themselves. This model, the "medical model" in health care, recognizes autonomy only on the part of the doctors, not the women-patients. Like the workplace model with technological control monopolized by management under the legal title of "managerial prerogative," the medical model emphasizes control from the top down, and expertise and competence in the hands of doctors and technicians, not the women. Furthermore, this model constantly reproduces itself — in the way most doctors are trained, most hospitals are run, and in the way individual pieces of technology are designed, manufactured and set up for daily use. Again, because these values and choices are built into the design and operating protocols of the technology, this gives the technology an almost deterministic quality. And to a certain extent this is part of its mystique, and deliberately cultivated as such: to appear as natural as women being confined to "traditional women's work" at a support-level status.

The deterministic inclinations are all man-made. But once the choices have been determined and set down in production, operating and education systems, they repeat themselves with a systemic dynamic as seemingly implacable as fate. Therefore, instead of there being a period of negotiation on how the experimental new reproductive technologies such as IVF should be introduced and used, their use is being patterned on the same old doctor-knows-best top-down orthodoxy of the entrenched medical model, with little or no opportunity for input on the part of women-users.

Patients are admitted only if they fit certain criteria, established and policed by the physicians running the clinic, which generally excludes lesbian couples and single women. Once the women are selected, their control over the techniques and technologies associated with AI, IVF and other treatments is limited to giving or withholding consent, based on limited information supplied by doctors in language which is often extremely difficult to understand (Stephens and McLean, 1993). The doctors assume (appropriate) the same "managerial prerogative" in their capacity as health-care professionals as management does in the workplace. Intrauterine insemination and AI are often accompanied by superovulation drugs (Stephens and McLean, 1993); yet unless the woman is infertile with an identifiable hormonal problem, there seems little reason to subject her to the risks, and costs, associated with fertility drugs.

On the other hand, there is the precedent of a Winnipeg AI program which sends out sperm by bus, packed in dry ice, to rural couples, who insert the sperm themselves (Stephens and McLean, 1993). While in some provinces insemination has been officially designated as a "delegated medical act" to be performed only by licensed professionals, in Manitoba technological users are still free to be technological practitioners, using techniques perfected by women over years of using tampons. So the system isn't necessarily closed.

The story of midwifery's comeback over the last 20 years offers us one of the best precedents for seeing how the production model approach to women's reproductive health can be overturned, and alternative technologies, such as techniques in assisting natural childbirth organized around women's physical and cultural priorities, can be put in place, even in mainstream hospitals.

There are also precedents in the area of physician-patient relationships. For instance, Dr. Jerilynn Prior of Vancouver is committed to an equal partnership between herself and her patients, and to the women having the final choice and say. In her research work on menopause, pre-menopause and factors affecting menstrual cycles, the women involved are collaborators in the research process (Prior, 1986), not passive objects or guinea pigs.

In the area of abortion, I have written elsewhere (Menzies, 1991) that if women could negotiate the use of abortion technology according to their own needs and priorities, they might organize the procedure so as to mitigate the pain and anguish many women suffer around this experience. Thus, a woman-defined abortion service might begin by acknowledging this pain, and provide some support in dealing with it as part of the abortion service. In addition to the technical-medical act, there might be a grieving ritual and opportunity for counselling and support from friends, peers and professionals.

The trouble is, there is little public discussion of these precedents. Or rather, they are part of another discourse on technology, one that is centred in women's actual experience, women's technological practice, not on technology divorced from the social context and on the officially designated experts. Meanwhile, the dominant or official discourse on abortion, as with other technologies, has been organized to virtually mirror the biases of the production model in the choice and organization of technology. It's organized as a debate for or against a given choice and organization of technology. Furthermore, it's a debate governed by designated experts, speaking the de-contextualized language of objective evidence and facts.

TECHNOLOGY AS DISCOURSE

A discussion Gwynne Basen, Abby Lippman and I have about IVF or pre-natal care around Margrit Eichler's kitchen table might pertain to the official discourse on the new reproductive technologies, but it's not likely to be recognized as part of it. The kind of discussion which is called "discourse" is usually a public discussion, and an officially designated and acknowledged one. It takes many institutional forms, such as academic texts and journals, encyclopedia and dictionaries. It also occurs through conferences organized by national and international institutions and official public inquiries such as the Royal Commission on the New Reproductive Technologies. Not just anyone gets to speak, or be heard, in this discussion, only those who are officially recognized as having something to say: generally, experts or "personal experience" witnesses who are, in turn, subject to cross-examination by the designated "commissioners" of the inquiry. The people who speak might contribute to the discussion, but they do not necessarily control it, nor its conclusions. It all depends on how the discussion is organized.

It's useful to think of discourse as a type of technological system — a cultural system of knowledge production rather than the more familiar material system producing and marketing things. We can ask, therefore, whether the discussion is open and democratic, with every participant contributing equally to its direction and outcome, or whether it's closed through pre-determined terms of reference governed and administered by some authority figure such as the chairperson of the Royal Commission on the New Reproductive Technologies?

Women's experience with the discourse on abortion since the 1960s is instructive. First, it wasn't a discourse created by women, but by men associated with medicine, law and the church. A 1986 study of how abortion was covered in the *Globe and Mail*, the Toronto *Star* and the Toronto *Sun* found that of the 760 sources quoted by these papers through 1986, two-thirds were men, and only one-third women. Of 66 people quoted in editorials in the *Globe and Mail*, only eight were women. Few pro- or anti-choice activists are quoted. Instead, the study found, the papers depend on doctors, lawyers and politicians — what it called "the elites" — as the main sources (Jones, 1990) and their focus was on the public-policy and medical issues, not personal experience.

Trying to represent women within the discourse, feminists were forced to adjust themselves to its overall structure: a debate for or against women's access to abortion as currently given — that is, as a procedure completely controlled by doctors acting as managers of the technology. The structure of the debate precluded discussing another way of organizing the technology, with women able to negotiate their use of it according to their personal needs and priorities. Furthermore, the language of the debate, the disembodied language of women's rights ("versus" so-called fetal rights) precluded talking about women's direct experience of abortion out of which a sense of women's actual needs could emerge. In addition to the abstract language, the polarized nature of the discourse styled as a debate kept women from testifying to the anguished choice which abortion represented to many women, lest they give ground to the other side in the debate. The silencing of this anguish not only aggravated many women's suffering. It also left women unsupported and alone in the hands of doctors who sometimes prolonged their pain and suffering in the way they treated them (Menzies, 1991 and Bowes, 1990).

Similar lessons can be drawn from the discourse on computer technology in the workplace, in which I myself was a participant through much of the 1980s. Here, too, the discussion was organized as a debate, a debate conducted by designated experts invited to speak at major national and international conferences. The debate was centred on "the long-term employment impacts of technology," with the choice, design and organization of the technology taken as given — and not open to discussion.

Increasingly, though, I found my thoughts and feelings returning to what workers whom I'd met had to say about organizing the technology differently. I started bringing these ideas into the official discourse, and trying to reframe the discussion around them. Then, I found myself increasingly marginalized, until finally, I wasn't invited to participate in the discussion at all.

Perhaps the lesson for us here is not to concentrate too much on trying to reform the official discourse. Perhaps the lesson is to ground ourselves in our own discourse. One that is consciously open and democratic, and centred in women's actual experience.

THE PERSONAL IS POLITICAL

For me, the positive and revolutionary part of the phrase "the personal is political" focuses on personal, lived experience, and how its evidence and example can change our society. It was by focusing on women's unpaid work in the home, and taking it seriously as work (not leisure and/or consumption), that Maggie Benston and other feminists made the breakthrough in thinking about women's liberation and women's work: that women's liberation would not be accomplished simply by women going out in the paid labour force and taking on the double burden of paid as well as unpaid work. It also requires that women's work in the home, the family and community be validated as productive labour (Benston, 1969).

With a similar focus on women's actual experience, feminist historians such as Jennifer Brown and Sylvia Van Kirk have revised conventional historical accounts — for instance, of the fur-trade period — by including women's conception of events, such as food preservation and translating from one language to another, and by including the women who did these things as bona fide historical agents. In science, feminists such as Margaret Alic have revised conventional understandings of what constitutes science by taking seriously the science women have done over the centuries, on their own terms. Building on and overlapping this, others such as Ursula Franklin and Maggie Benston have opened the frame of reference to welcome a broader range of inquiry and activity, including a lot of the citizen science and grassroots science which women continue to do in the community and in the peace, environmental and other activist movements.

Likewise, it was by focusing on women's actual experience, as telephone operators and office workers, that I could break out of the mould of the official discourse on technology in the workplace, with its limited options of being for or against a particular choice and organization of technology (Menzies, 1989). It was by taking these women seriously as technological practitioners that I could begin to see another option: that of organizing the technology their way — which tended to be in ways that enlarged and extended public service and didn't just automate what services were presently provided. Similarly, it was by focusing on women's actual experience with abortion that I was able to see how the feminist discussion on abortion could and even must move beyond the limits set by the official discourse: namely, women's access to safe abortions. Women don't just need access to the technology. We need to be able to control it. And there's no reason why we can't — given the precedents I mentioned earlier.

The feminist discourse on the new reproductive technologies is just beginning. This book demystifies the technology and offers a preliminary analysis of it. The next step is to stimulate an open, democratic discussion about women's reproductive health, out of which a sense of the appropriate choice, place and organization of various technologies will hopefully emerge. If the personal is political, then an open, inclusive discussion in which every woman's experience is recognized as valid and true, will yield an open, inclusive approach to the goal of empowering women to have healthy babies and healthy sex lives with the minimum of intervention and related dependency.

I trust the process, and invite you to do so too.

ACKNOWLEDGMENT

I wish to thank Janice McLean for valuable comments on an early draft of this chapter.

SOURCES

Alic, Margaret, 1986. *Hypatia's Heritage: A History of Women in Science from Antiquity through the Nineteenth Century*. Boston: Beacon Hill Press.

Benston, Maggie, 1969. "The political economy of women's liberation," *Monthly Review*, 1969. See also Angela Miles's article on this work in *Canadian Woman Studies/les cahiers de la femme*, Vol. 13, No. 2.

Benston, Maggie, 1993. In conversation with Ursula Franklin, "Complexity and management," *Canadian Woman Studies/les cahiers de la femme*, 66.

Bowes, Nancy, 1990. *Telling our Secrets: Abortion Stories from Nova Scotia*, Halifax: CARAL.

Eisler, Riane, 1988. *The Chalice and the Blade*, San Francisco, Harper & Row.

Franklin, Ursula, 1990. *The Real World of Technology*, Toronto: Anansi Press.

Jones, Deborah, 1990. "Ignoring the ethics of abortion?" *The Globe and Mail*, June 8.

Jones, Laura & Davidson, Eileen, 1990. Dalkon Shield Action Canada brief to Royal Commission on New Reproductive Technologies, Ottawa.

MacDonald, Marilyn, 1987. Private conversation.

Menzies, Heather, 1989. *Fastforward and Out of Control*, Toronto: MacMillan of Canada.

    1991. "Rethinking abortion," *Canadian Forum*, October.

Prior, Jerilynn C., 1986. "The therapy of reproductive system changes associated with exercise training," *The Menstrual Cycle and Physical Activity*, eds. J. Puhl & H.Brown, Champagne, Illinois: Human Kinetics Publishers.

Rauhala, Ann, 1987. "Despite dangers, 1.5 million Canadians take birth-control pills," The *Globe and Mail*, Oct. 13.

Rennie, Susan, 1993. "Breast cancer prevention: Diet vs. drugs," *Ms. Magazine*, Vol. III, No. 6.

Simand, Harriet, 1990. DES Action/Canada brief to Royal Commission on New Reproductive Technologies, Ottawa.

Stephens, Thomas & McLean, Janice, *1993. Survey of Canadian Fertility Programs*, Ottawa: Royal Commission on the New Reproductive Technologies.

NOTES

1   "In his Image: Science and Technology as Ideology," *This Magazine*, May/June, 1987.

2   The word engineer derives from the latin word *genere*, which means to sire; the male role in procreation.

3   Re-member means to put together again, to rejoin pieces of things, and bodies, which have broken apart. The word is used here to deliberately evoke a bodily and organic sense of women remembering.

4   In October, 1992, Harvard University researcher Walter Willett concluded that women whose dietary fat averaged 29 percent had the same incidence of breast cancer as those with 49 percent fat, and that this evidence should be taken as settling the debate about diet and breast cancer. However, a low-fat diet is considered to be one with less than 20 percent fat, not less than 30 percent (Rennie, 1993)

17

Kate Fillion

"God isn't going to get you pregnant, the doctor is going to get you pregnant," says Lynne Martin. (Names and identifying details of all infertility patients and their doctors have been changed to protect privacy.) Her husband, John, says, "Every month for three days it's like a funeral. We've had twenty-four funerals. If she does get pregnant, I'm not going to feel that something is beginning. I'm going to feel 'Thank God it's over.'"

Six-thirty a.m., early July, the waiting room of a Toronto clinic that specializes in fertility drugs and artificial insemination. It's a no-frills operation compared to the virtual shopping malls for reproductive miracles that offer everything from microsurgery to *in vitro* fertilization. Already twenty patients, all women, are here: financiers, nurses, bank tellers, lawyers, teachers from all over Ontario. Some get up at 4 to drive to the clinic; others live so far away they fly in for treatment. They range in age from mid-20s to mid-40s, but the majority are between 36 and 40; most have been trying to get pregnant for four to six years.

Usually there's a bleary-eyed camaraderie among the women, who know the intimate details of each other's menstrual cycles and reproductive heartbreak. They swap information on doctors, console one another about sluggish ovaries and their husband's sperm counts, and joke about the rigours of sex on demand.

Today, however, the mood borders on mutinous. It started when a no-nonsense blonde snapped, "I want a consult with Dr. — but my own doctor seems reluctant. Maybe his feelings are hurt but too bad! He's not aggressive enough, he has 5,000 patients —" A ripple of astonishment: 5,000? "Yes! How can he keep track of us all? I got pregnant in the fall of '88, then had a miscarriage. Here we are, 1991. I'm tired of waiting."

There's a whiplash of discomfort — *you don't want to rock the boat, it might jeopardize your treatment* — while discontent snakes around the room: the bathroom is filthy, there are no sheets in the examination rooms on weekends, a sperm wash costs $100 here but only $90 at another clinic. And the scheduling problems! Like most clinics, this one operates on a first-come, first-served basis; women start arriving long before the 7 a.m. opening and take numbers, hoping to finish in time for work.

The key to most infertility treatments is close monitoring of — and often pharmaceutical control over — ovulation, when the egg is released from its follicle (a sort of holding sack) and for the next twenty-four hours is ripe for fertilization. Maximizing that narrow window of reproductive opportunity requires daily blood tests to measure key hormone levels and vaginal ultrasounds to track the growth of follicles. The wait for the ten-minute tests averages an hour and a half but can be much longer on busy days.

At noon, patients return to receive the results, which, if they're on fertility drugs, determine the day's dosage. Right around the time of ovulation they're inseminated with their partner's or a donor's sperm, usually on two subsequent days, at which point clinic visits cease and they wait to find out if they're pregnant. The process typically lasts a week but can take longer, depending on the length of a woman's menstrual cycle and the drugs prescribed.

"I'm almost at the end of my rope," one woman says. "You wait hours, get jabbed with needles, someone shoves an ultrasound probe inside you, then you come back in the afternoon and a doctor squirts sperm in. It's starting to feel very intrusive."

These are not minor complaints, but the major ones go unspoken: *Why, with all this technological wizardry, aren't we getting pregnant? What's the matter with us?*

For many, it's the first time they've failed at anything. They did the difficult things — climbing the career ladder, buying a home — with such ease that it seems ridiculous that this easy thing, reproduction, is so very difficult. After those shock-tactic lectures — *just a few minutes in the backseat of a car, girls, that's all it takes* — all that talk about *controlling* fertility, *planning* a family, as if conception were an act of will. After being responsible and waiting for the right time, finally throwing out the contraceptives and, oh God! those proud we've-decided-to-start-a-family announcements — isn't it supposed to just happen? *I feel out of control,* they say again and again.

Science seems to offer the opportunity to take charge of reproductive destiny: find the best doctor, the newest treatment, the hottest drugs, the most state-of-the-art equipment, and you can conquer biology!

The quest for the right baby-making formula is as seductive as it is unerotic. Success is no further away than the clinic's bulletin board, studded with baby photos and heartfelt notes from new parents.

Who could object to embracing technology to satisfy the most natural human urge? It would be easy to answer if the implications were limited to cuddly newborns, but there are also scientific, legal and moral implications, so complex they make the abortion issue look simple.

Forget Darwinism: postmenopausal women now bear children, scientists "help" incompetent sperm penetrate eggs, embryos are frozen and thawed and tested for hundreds of chromosomal abnormalities. Doctors talk of "recruiting" and "harvesting" eggs, "washing" and "banking" sperm, "running" menstrual cycles and "reducing" embryos. The day is not far off when advances in genetic technologies will make it possible to manipulate the biological makeup of humans when they are merely clusters of cells in a petri dish.

The simplest question is whether the new reproductive technologies (NRTs) are medically benign. The answer is that no one really knows. Almost all advanced treatments, including *in vitro* fertilization (IVF) and related laboratory procedures, require drugs for which there have been few related randomized trials.

Doctors argue that some have been prescribed for years, without apparent problems: no news is good news. However, there are virtually no studies of the long-term effects on women and children, which is worrying given the tragic history of drugs prescribed during pregnancy: thalidomide and DES, to name two. There were no randomized trials of DES, a synthetic estrogen prescribed from 1941 to 1971; its disastrous results — cancer and reproductive failure in offspring — didn't show up for years.

Informed consent is tricky as real information about risks is scarce and clinics have no standard definition of success: Is it chemical pregnancy? Or a fetal heartbeat? Or a birth? Or a healthy "take-home" baby? At best, the information given to patients is difficult to interpret and at worst, deliberately misleading. For instance, IVF clinics claim twenty to thirty percent success rates when in fact their results measured in terms of live births are between zero and thirteen percent, according to a 1988 survey by Ann Pappert, a Toronto writer who's extensively researched NRTs. Despite less than overwhelming results, procedures like IVF are used increasingly, which has led to questions about their real purpose: making babies or advancing science?

"The new reproductive technologies have been presented as a solution to infertility, and I think that's a smoke screen. Something like IVF, with a failure rate of ninety percent, would not normally be accepted as a medical treatment," says Toronto sociology professor Margrit Eichler. "It may incidentally be useful to a few infertile couples, but in my view, the main reason IVF is done is to generate 'surplus' embryos, which permit genetic research."

The future applications of the whiz-bang genetic technologies that are developing in tandem with the NRTs are indeed troubling. Applying industrial and engineering principles to reproduction — creating the embryo, quality controlling it, screening it for defects — raises the spectre of made-to-order babies. Now the focus is on eliminating disease, but when does the therapeutic intervention become eugenics? In the not-so-distant future, who will decide whether an embryo with a fifty-fifty chance of developing a crippling disorder should be implanted? Or whether a gene for, say, green eyes is desirable or not?

"If you have a personal, individual encounter with the technology, it doesn't seem sinister," says Varda Burstyn, until recently the NRT spokeswoman for the National Action Committee on the Status of Women (NAC). "But if you step up from the level of the individual and look at the social aggregate, you get a very different impression. I don't judge any woman for wanting to have a child and possibly doing anything she can to have one, but I sure do judge medical scientists and pharmaceutical companies — which are the driving forces behind these technologies — for putting into her path a technology that is dangerous to her health and *wildly* ineffective, which she will nevertheless want to try because of her desire to have children."

NAC's call for rigorous scrutiny of existing NRTs, with no further expansion until the verdict is in, is explosively controversial. Many in the medical community dismiss critics of the NRTs as scaremongers; scientists argue that the "extra" embryos created by the NRTs permit research that may provide a cure for any number of diseases.

And back in the waiting room, the weary predawn conviviality gives way to bristling irony at the very suggestion of a moratorium: *Excuse me, don't women have the right to make their own reproductive choices? I want to be here — I tried to get bumped up on the waiting list, for God's sake — I'll do anything to have baby! What does pro-choice mean, anyway?*

One of these women is Emma Dixon, who's in her first week of infertility treatment. This debate seems far removed from her own life. She's not thinking about genetic engineering but about babies, the baby she wants, and she's hopeful, so hopeful she's agreed to let me tag along in the mornings. Over the next nine months, I become a sort of reproductive cheerleader, rooting for a happy ending. Partly for Emma, of course, and partly because if the trade-off for the unpleasantness, potential risks and possible future uses of the NRTs is a baby, then there is at least one easy answer to some very complicated questions of ends and means.

"Infertility is a major, major problem in this country," says Dr. Michael Virro, an infertility specialist at Markham-Stouffville Hospital.

End of consensus. The definition, extent and causes of infertility are all hotly debated, as are treatment methods. Infertility used to be seen as a judgment from God, a stigma; usually the woman was blamed, and "treatment" consisted of divorce, adoption or childlessness. Attitudes have changed dramatically since the advent of NRTs, so it's unclear whether infertility is actually increasing or there are simply more couples seeking treatment.

Many of the "infertile" are actually not sterile but subfertile: capable of conceiving without medical intervention but with more than average difficulty. Sometimes couples who easily conceived one child experience secondary infertility; those seeking to reverse voluntary sterility after a tubal ligation or vasectomy are also considered infertile.

For couples not using contraception, the chances of getting pregnant in any given cycle are fifteen to twenty percent: these odds are not cumulative and remain the same every month. If infertility is defined as failure to conceive after twelve months of unprotected sex, roughly twenty percent of all couples are infertile. If the deadline is extended to eighteen months, the figure drops to ten percent.

Medical remedies are being tested and refined so rapidly that specialists must scramble to keep up. There is, however, a fairly standard continuum of treatment: monitoring a woman's natural menstrual cycle to calibrate intercourse to ovulation, then insemination with a partner's or donor's "washed" (purified) sperm, next coupling artificial insemination with a range of progressively more powerful fertility drugs, and finally combining these drugs with laboratory procedures such as IVF to try to control scientifically the meeting of egg and sperm.

Although it's still a matter of intense speculation, thirty-five percent of infertility is believed to be related to male factors, thirty-five percent to female factors, twenty percent to combined male and female factors, and ten percent is unexplained. Sometimes there's a physiological reason, such as blocked or scarred fallopian tubes, in some cases the cause being a sexually transmitted disease. Experts forecast a future increase in infertility due to chlamydia, an often symptomless STD that's currently rampant among teens, which can lead to pelvic inflammatory disease. Most often, however, the problem is either a low sperm count or, for women, irregular ovulation.

And then there's age. Men, as a former prime minister demonstrated recently, can become fathers in their 70s. For women, on the other hand, it becomes markedly and increasingly more difficult to get pregnant — and carry a chromosomally normal baby to term — after the age of 34.

Over the past thirty years, the median age of first-time mothers has crept steadily upwards. In 1961, only sixteen percent of babies born to Canadian women in their late 30s were first or second children; by 1989, it was 37.5 percent. And whereas in 1961 two-thirds of the babies born to women in their early 40s were at least fifth children, today almost half are first or second children.

"The bottom line is that if women had babies in their 20s and focused on their careers in their 30s, we wouldn't have as many infertility problems," says Dr. Virro. "But I don't think you shouldn't treat a woman just because she's over 40 — enough 42- and 43-year-olds get pregnant."

Emma Dixon, 40, and her husband Ian, 39, are successful professionals in fields with relatively modest economic rewards. She is warmly wry and delicately attractive, he's a cheerful skeptic with boyish charm. After their marriage (her first, his second) two and a half years ago, they began trying to have a baby.

"Although I get angry when people say that just because I'm a woman and I'm 40, I'm too old to have a baby, sometimes I think of it the same way," Emma said last July. "I'll be 60 when the child is 20 — can I cope with that?"

"Emma thinks I'll be really depressed if we don't get pregnant, but part of me would feel liberated," Ian said separately. "At the moment my career is on hold, I can't quit my job, because we'll need the security if we have a baby. And the neurotic side of me thinks I'd be a shitty father, because I don't really know aside from movies and books what a good parent does. So I'm still somewhat ambivalent and yet, when I see men with their kids in the park, it's immensely painful. I want that sense of connection."

When they stopped using birth control, Emma's GP had her chart her basal body temperature, which entailed sticking a thermometer in her mouth every morning before she got up and graphing the minute fluctuations. A drop in temperature followed by a sustained rise heralds ovulation; couples are advised to have sex every forty-eight hours just prior to, during and after ovulation.

"You're only supposed to use certain positions, then lie on your back with a pillow under your hips for about half an hour," groans Emma. "One morning I woke up with a bad cold and had to wake Ian, who is not a morning person, and say, 'We've got to do it now.' It was horrid. We decided we wouldn't do that again, this is not how we want to make a baby, it has to be something aside from a mere performance."

Emma at first "just assumed" she'd get pregnant. "Certainly I've had many disappointments in life, but usually if I want something enough I get it. I didn't think it would take that much work." As the months passed, they became puzzled, then anxious. Emma, very svelte, gained some weight hoping it would help her conceive, and began to wonder if somehow she was being punished. Perhaps she'd been too blithe about conception, she'd taken the Pill and used an IUD — what had that done to her system? Or had she simply waited too long? Ian had smoked pot back when everyone did — was that the problem?

"You become so focused on this one thing you can't do. I hate myself for thinking like this, but I started to feel I was failing as a woman," says Emma. "I see a pregnant woman — I don't know her, don't know what her life is like, but I hate her. Just seeing a child can make me teary."

She wasn't alone. "At the squash club a friend told me his wife was pregnant," Ian remembers. "He said, 'We've got lots of time to have a second one after this.' I said, 'I'm so happy for you.' But I'm thinking, The bastard! Wait till we get on the court, I'll whip your ass. It's competitive, like you have to *earn* it, have the pain and difficulty before we'll be happy for you."

After six months Emma's GP reviewed her temperature charts, announced she wasn't ovulating regularly, and asked, "Would it be devastating if you didn't get pregnant?" The possibility had never even occurred to Emma. "I felt this pit open in my stomach and realized, My God, I really do want children. I started to cry and the doctor said, 'This is no time to get emotional.'"

Within two months — "incredibly quickly" — the Dixons had an appointment with Dr. Roger Owen at an infertility clinic. There was a battery of blood tests to measure their respective hormone levels and rule out infections; Ian's semen and Emma's cervical mucus were analyzed. Then Emma had a laparoscopy, a surgical procedure that determines whether a woman's pelvic organs are normal. Dr. Owen detected endometriosis (a disease in which the lining of the uterus migrates to other organs, often causing scarring and blockages that lead to fertility problems), and removed it with a laser. Had eleven months of scheduling sex with military precision been squandered?

When he went over the test results, Dr. Owen struck them both as less than approachable. "His attitude is, You don't need to understand this, just trust me," says Ian. "And he's far more sensitive to me in some ways than to Emma. He was very matter of fact about her endometriosis and irregular menstruation, but turned on all his most sensitive charm in breaking the sad news that on one occasion I had a low sperm count. It's so silly, but I responded in exactly the same way Sylvester Stallone would. I wanted to say, 'Let me do it again, I'll show you!'"

Dr. Owen proposed that after a diagnostic cycle to monitor Emma's natural ovulation, fertility drugs were the ticket. When women ovulate, they normally release one egg. The idea behind ova-stimulating drugs is to regulate ovulation and increase the number of eggs and thus the chances that at least one will fertilize and result in a pregnancy. The drugs most commonly used are Clomid, which spurs ovulation and "recruits" more than one egg per cycle, and Pergonal, a powerful hormone that pushes follicles to mature.

Emma was wary. She hates needles — Pergonal is injected deep into the hip muscle, often several times daily — and had heard about the extreme mood swings, abdominal pain and hot flashes that are common side effects. *It seems that if we're meant to have a baby, we shouldn't have to do this.*

They asked about the drugs' long-term effects. Dr. Owen said they were completely safe but, he allowed, there was an increased chance of multiple births. In fact, about five percent of pregnancies result in three or more fetuses; twenty to twenty-five percent of women who get pregnant on the drugs have multiple births.

"Don't worry about triplets, we can reduce the embryos," the doctor soothed. Selective reduction, in which potassium chloride is injected directly into the thorax of a targeted fetus to stop its heart, is usually performed only when fetal abnormalities are detected or the number of fetuses endangers the pregnancy. It is, obviously, controversial; sometimes "reduction" is tragically unselective and the woman loses the pregnancy altogether. *What are we doing, making a baby or killing one?*

The Dixons resolved not to think about the drugs until they had to. After all, Dr. Owen said they had a twenty percent chance of conceiving on a monitored drug-free cycle. Or was it fifteen percent? Or less? Or had that twenty percent chance been *with* drugs? There had been so many numbers flying around the office that neither of them could remember for sure. Like most couples new to fertility treatment, it never occurred to them to ask how many of those pregnancies resulted in live births. *The doctors talk about success rates, and you assume they mean babies. How is a miscarriage a success?*

Well, whatever. *The guy's an expert and if he lacks warmth, isn't that just what all specialists are like?* Emma, arms aching from the morning blood tests and exhausted from racing between her office and the clinic, was determined to be positive. *At least we're finally doing something.* But during the afternoon appointment when Dr. Owen went over the morning's results, she was acutely aware of the other women tapping their feet in the waiting room and too intimidated to ask questions. *He's so busy, by the time I think of what I want to ask, he's out the door. That's one problem I have with this process, no one ever tells you exactly what's going on.*

After eight days, it was time for Emma's first intrauterine insemination: "washed," or purified, sperm are injected through a catheter directly into the uterus. Couples are generally advised to abstain from intercourse around the time of ovulation, to improve the odds of a good semen sample. The procedure was the closest Emma and Ian got to sex for days, and left him visibly shaken: "I tried to fantasize in the washroom at work, then rushed over with the sample. We go into the examination room and Emma takes her clothes off, Dr. Owen runs in and looks at the sperm under the microscope then turns around, smiles, and gestures for her to spread her legs." Ian holds his palms together as if praying, then lowers them as if parting the Red Sea.

"God, the doctor's gesture bothered me! She obediently spread her legs — it's all a blur, I'm standing against the wall — and he starts talking about his new car while shoving a cold speculum into her, at which point she flinches and I want to hit him. My reaction was very primal: I'm thinking, *Who is this guy fondling my wife?* It's a very intimate thing and I had no part in it. When he injected the sperm he kind of smirked, 'Oh yeah, now we should have some romantic music' — there was no acknowledgment that this is an emotional as well as a biological moment. The atmosphere is rush, rush, rush, no questions because another couple's waiting, the doctor's excited about his new car... you feel like a small part of this big machine."

Ian didn't want to go to the second insemination, but Emma insisted. She was used to being "poked and prodded" and needed to feel they were in this together. The next day, clutching his semen sample in a brown paper bag, Ian was doubtfully plucky: "We've made love when Emma's ovulating and it's been intensely exciting. It had never occurred to me to say, I can transfer that feeling and this clinical experience could be seen as powerful."

Later they were upbeat. "At the very least this technology is telling me I'm ovulating and I feel better knowing my body is doing what it should. And maybe I'm pregnant!" Emma beamed at Ian, then looked stricken. "Oh God, maybe I shouldn't think that, it will be more devastating if I'm not. I'm just going to block it out."

But being pregnant was all she could think about. She worried — *Is it okay to have a glass of wine? What about coffee?* — and then worried that worrying would somehow jinx the process. She felt elation, then fear: *What if it didn't work and I have to take the drugs? No, better think positive. Or is thinking positively just an invitation for failure?*

Two weeks later, her period didn't arrive on schedule. Neither she nor Ian said anything for a day. By the second night, they were lying in bed, talking tentatively about the baby that might be, feeling blessed. It had been worth it, the inconvenience and the discomfort and the coldness of it all.

The next day, she got her period.

Reproductive biology was a decidedly unglamorous specialty until 1978, when Louise Brown, the world's first baby conceived *in vitro* (literally, "in glass"), was born. *In vitro* fertilization is all about trying to beat the odds. Fertility drugs are used aggressively to create as many eggs as possible; if they fertilize when combined in a petri dish with sperm, multiple embryos are generally implanted in a woman's uterus, to improve the chances that one will "take" and result in a viable pregnancy. This is why so many IVF pregnancies result in multiple births. And the drive to create as many embryos as possible means there are "leftovers," which can be frozen, given to other infertile couples or donated to research.

IVF generated a cottage industry for social commentators. A miracle cure for infertility! No, an open door for genetic engineering! But research on artificially created embryos may deliver a cancer cure! Maybe, but it's morally wrong to create life outside the body! Legal experts pondered hypothetical questions that soon became realities: who "owns" frozen embryos if a couple divorces or both die? Others wondered about the ethics of experimenting on embryos: Is it tantamount to experimentation on humans?

Many of the dilemmas remain unresolved and now there are new ones, due to a virtual explosion in reproductive medicine. New reproductive and genetic technologies are making it possible to manipulate genes at the earliest stage of life, and they're proliferating in a moral vacuum.

Already, IVF is big business. Initially, the technique was used primarily for women with blocked fallopian tubes, but clinics now accept couples with many other fertility problems, although success rates haven't improved for six years. In some clinics, more women on the waiting list get pregnant, with no treatment whatsoever, than those who actually undergo IVF. In medical terms, the World Health Organization argues, it is a failed technology.

Low success rates aren't the only problem. Women who undergo IVF are considerably more likely to have miscarriages and ectopic pregnancies, a potentially life-threatening condition in which the embryo grows outside the uterus and must be aborted. And in 1988, Australia — the only country in the world that assiduously tracks IVF babies and their mothers — released a disturbing preliminary report of its registry. The results: the chances of having a baby through IVF are 8.8 percent, but the odds of having a *live, healthy* baby are only 4.8 percent. IVF babies are five times as likely to have spina bifida and seven times more likely to have transposed heart vessels.

Other studies have shown that neonatal and perinatal mortality rates are much higher for IVF babies. And, primarily because of the high incidence of multiple births, IVF babies have over eleven times the rate of low birth weight, which is associated with a host of long-term developmental problems.

If the health risks associated with IVF are drug related — without studies, who knows? — then there are implications for *all* women who take fertility drugs. Some researchers believe the genetic abnormalities that have been documented in twenty percent of IVF embryos may have something to do with ova-stimulating drugs. But no one really knows for sure.

The drugs are otherworldly (Pergonal is made from the urine of post-menopausal Italian nuns), extremely expensive, and in many cases, what passes for research on them is really a collection of recipes: clinic A got twenty pregnancies using Pergonal, clinic B got twenty-two pregnancies with Pergonal and Clomid. The only absolutely proven serious health risk is the hyperstimulation syndrome: in two percent of women who take ova-stimulating drugs, the ovaries become dangerously enlarged and fluid accumulates in the abdomen and/or lungs.

But some drugs haven't been used in the NRTs long enough even to make long-term studies possible. One is Lupron, an extremely powerful drug generally used to suppress a woman's natural menstrual cycle, in effect inducing a sort of menopause. With other drugs to grow eggs and induce ovulation, doctors can then completely control her reproductive system.

"The absolute safety of Lupron won't be determined for two generations, but I think it's very safe if properly monitored, and the half-life is very short," says Dr. Alan Shewchuk, whose infertility clinic is affiliated with Toronto Hospital. "People with reproductive failure have an inherently higher risk of having kids with congenital abnormalities. Is this a result of the drugs or the health problems the patient has in association with not getting pregnant? You need massive studies for statistical significance. Let's put it this way: if my daughter were 35 and had endometriosis, I wouldn't hesitate to use Lupron."

Others are less sanguine. French IVF guru Jacques Testart told Ann Pappert, who is writing a book on IVF, that "he and many of the people on his IVF team were deeply concerned about the increased risk of cancer from [Lupron and similar drugs].[1] When I asked Testart why, then, the drugs continue to be used, he replied that scientists were learning a great deal about conception, and this was of vital importance."

Given the connections between estrogen and breast cancer, there are serious concerns about possible long-term effects of the "hormonal cocktails" served up in infertility treatments. Will they cause premature menopause? Ovarian cancer? Are the rumours from Australia about increased rates of childhood cancer true?[2]

Canada certainly won't be supplying any answers. Only now is a voluntary registry being established (with start-up funds from Serono, the pharmaceutical giant in the lucrative infertility industry) so that clinics can record success rates. Voluntary, however, is the operative word: doctors were reluctant, or even refused, to supply statistics even for the Royal Commission on The New Reproductive Technologies, for its survey on Canadian Fertility Programs, published in May, 1993. Ontario, the only province in Canada — and one of the few governments in the world — that fully funds IVF in hospital-based clinics, has no guidelines for drug usage or even limits on the number of embryos that can be implanted per cycle.[3]

The most conservative estimate is that one IVF baby costs taxpayers $40,000, based on one in ten of the $4,000 procedures succeeding. However, that figure does *not* include the costs of many of the diagnostic and monitoring tests, or the mother's obstetrical care, or the neonatal intensive care that an unusually large proportion of IVF babies require. Nor does it reflect the costs to individual couples: time off work while going through the all-consuming program, fertility drugs ($1,000 to $2,000 per cycle, which many insurance companies will not cover), or the minimum $3,000 per cycle charged in private clinics. And it certainly doesn't include any of the long-term costs associated with low birth weight and preterm births, which are common in IVF because of the high percentage of multiple births.

The real figure is probably closer to $100,000 per baby, but the province doesn't appear terribly interested in tracking what it's getting for the millions of dollars spent on IVF or the other infertility treatments offered in the dozen clinics in the Metro area. Although the previous Liberal government did commission a study on IVF clinics, it's never been released. "It's an interministerial report," says Ministry of Health spokesman Layne Verbeek. "It's still under review."

When former Health Minister Frances Lankin announced that the government was considering cuts to IVF funding, there was a predictable outcry about the spectre of a two-tiered health care system. In fact, infertility clinics *are* two-tiered: the poor are not lining up to have more children. However, politicians are wary of cutting funding because infertility treatments seem politically correct: pro-family, pro-reproductive freedom.

Couples who demand access frame the issue in terms of personal choice. "There is nothing that we will not do to have our own child," one man in his 40s told the Royal Commission on The New Reproductive Technologies. "We have done everything conceivable, followed every avenue of technology for fifteen years.... If technology gives us a chance of having a child, which I believe we are entitled to, please, let us have that opportunity."

Many argue that public funding is appropriate because the anguish of infertility is as debilitating as that caused by a disease. "Infertility is an illness as far as I'm concerned, and there are risks with every drug you take for any illness," says Sarah Dallon, who recently had quadruplets as a result of fertility drugs, after trying to conceive for five years. "When the doctor said, 'I'm going to get you pregnant,' I knew there were some serious risks, but at that point I would have tried anything."

Many couples feel they are the only ones who can make an accurate cost-benefit analysis. As one new father testified to the RCNRT, "My wife was fully informed of the risks of fertility therapies and unfortunately, unusually prone to their side effects. She got sweats, cramps, spells of depression, just outbursts of crying in the middle of the night, atrophy of the vagina, including painful cracking of the labia. Of course, there was the poking and prodding.... Only she can say if it was worth it, and she believes it was."

The problem for the public health system is that medical advances are occurring so rapidly that many couples simply will not give up the baby quest. One new technique makes it possible for postmenopausal women to become pregnant — Where should the line be drawn, and by whom? If a man has a low sperm count, should taxpayers foot the bill for fifteen years of infertility treatments for his wife if they don't want to try donor sperm or adoption?

For those couples who succeed, the upside of infertility treatments is very clear. But even doctors agree that their vocal and enthusiastic defence gives a somewhat skewed impression of the medical efficacy of the NRTs.

"The way infertility clinics work is that a third of our patients get pregnant *in spite* of us, just from better reproductive hygiene. A third get pregnant because of us, as a direct result of what we do. And another third won't get pregnant," says Dr. Shewchuk. "So two-thirds think we're pretty bright, and tell their ten friends, and this thing just keeps repeating itself. Patients have to understand that no infertility clinic in the world works magic. Sure, some miracles do happen here, but we are not miracle workers."

It's September, Emma's first day back in the clinic. Like many patients, she took August off to go on vacation. She's decided to do another drug-free monitored cycle. "I know this sounds crazy but I really don't want a drug-induced baby, it just seems that much more removed from us."

She emerges from the ultrasound exam looking as if she'd like to throttle Dr. Owen. "I'm already ovulating. That means I only get one insemination, not two. Damn it!"

She's keenly aware that she has a limited number of chances left, and if she never does get pregnant, she'll look back on this one insemination, this half-chance, and wonder, *What if?* There are many younger and thus "more suitable" would-be parents already waiting to adopt. Nor would Emma be a good candidate even for the last-ditch gamble of IVF; the success rate for women over 39 is so negligible that most hospital clinics, where waiting lists are already long, will not accept them.

"I don't feel old and yet, in terms of this process, I am," she says. "That has been a huge emotional hurdle for me. Maybe I should have been trying to have a baby when I was 30, but I hadn't met Ian, I wasn't ready.... Maybe I should have organized my priorities a little differently."

But society told her: you can control your fertility; you can have sex and not wind up barefoot and pregnant. It's a terrible irony for women of her generation to find out that perhaps biology is destiny, after all; their contraceptive freedom may seem in retrospect to have been something of a trap. Many of these trailblazers who redefined women's roles revert to the stereotypes they overthrew when describing their inability to conceive: I feel I've failed as a woman because I can't be a mother.

If I had had fewer choices, Emma thinks, *I might not be in this position. So, do I wish I hadn't had those choices or made the decisions I did?*

Dr. Alan Shewchuk is a legendary baby-maker, and looks the part: white coat, silver hair and a rumbling Marcus Welby voice that lulls you into an all's-well-with-the-world state while he draws diagrams of the molecular structure of fertility drugs.

Wreathed in smoke, he attaches orange stickers to the files stacked on his desk. "Orange is for the pregnancies. I've got to get one pregnancy a day," he says. "It's like a crossword puzzle. I work very hard on the numbers; we do incredibly detailed workups here."

His reputation means a long waiting list and a full waiting room. "It's a zoo," one of his patients grumbled. He smiles avuncularly when I repeat this. "The wait isn't really longer than at the hairdresser's. Most of my patients take the week off work and loaf through the program. They come in later, do their blood and ultrasound, go do their shopping, meet the girls for brunch, come back in the afternoon, go see a movie, then go home and get tidied up, and the husband comes and picks them up and takes them out to dinner. There's less stress."

Lynne Martin, 28, laughs at the notion that anyone could loaf through an infertility program. She's a nurse, so she knows all about the failings of the human body, and three years of infertility have convinced her that sometimes the pain you can't see is the worst. "Every time I get my period, I've lost control, and hope, and a dream," she says. "I feel so alone sometimes that I just want to crawl into the closet, some tiny enclosed space somewhere, and never come out."

She's taken fertility drugs on and off for two years; last year her husband, John, 30, underwent an operation to repair a varicocele, a varicose vein of the scrotum, in a successful attempt to improve his sperm count.

Even if Lynne could take time off work while undergoing treatment, it would hardly be stress-free. "My emotions are all over the map because of the drugs, my bum aches from the injection. After the insemination the progesterone suppositories make my breasts hurt and I have hot flashes. I can't trust my body any more, it's sending me all these signs that I'm pregnant and I don't know whether I really am or it's just the drugs. During the twelve days of hell waiting to see if it's going to work, sex is really painful because my ovaries are so swollen with eggs. I can't have a cup of tea or a glass of wine because I might be pregnant, and now I can't even have a normal sexual relationship with my husband, which is more important than ever. You just feel crummy for two weeks, and then get your period and feel crummy about that. You go through a grieving process; you think, what good am I?"

Worse than the physical side effects was the initial strain on her marriage. "Lynne was upset because at first, I didn't give her unconditional support," says John, a pull-no-punches kind of guy. "She was always worrying — Is this going to work? What if it doesn't? — on and on. I did not subscribe to her emotional fallout, the funeral every month. It was as though a close friend of hers, who I'd never met, had died. All I saw was her anguish and grief. My feelings were primarily a reaction to hers."

Now their biggest worries are financial. Her insurance plan won't cover more fertility drugs, and John's company decides on a month-by-month basis whether to continue paying. Lynne, terrified she'll be cut off, has started stockpiling Pergonal — even if they invest $10,000 of their own, it only would buy a five-month supply and no guarantees. At this point she'd gladly gamble. "Lynne will do anything, short of kidnapping, to have a child," says John.

She'd be prepared to adopt but, like many men in infertile couples, John is more reluctant. One issue seems to be that adoption entails someone else judging their fitness for parenthood; infertility treatment requires no home studies or psychological assessments, nor are men involved in most of it. Waiting lists are also very long, and private adoption can be costly, not to mention reversible if the birth mother changes her mind. So, says Lynne attempting perkiness, she'll probably continue treatment for a few more years. God willing. Or God forbid.

"I'm beginning to wonder how far we should go. The issue gets clouded because of personal desire, you lose sight of the intellectual questions because you're so driven by what you want. For the past three years I've thought about having a baby. Every single day. We are put on this earth to reproduce and I really want to be pregnant, I want the experience. Each cycle is a new beginning, a new chance, it feels like you're doing something active to achieve your goal, and it feels so good to hope, it's like infatuation. But that's the problem — you get addicted to hope."

Many doctors also seem unwilling to write off losses. There's tremendous competition among infertility specialists; they all want to be seen as the best, and many of their theories are diametrically opposed. Gamete intrafallopian transfer (GIFT) is a good example. The procedure is similar to IVF except eggs are not fertilized outside the body; rather they're placed together with sperm in the fallopian tubes, where fertilization normally occurs.

"Without a doubt, the most stupid procedure," Dr. Shewchuk gently scoffs. "You'll get a high success rate if you select your patients, but you will not get a higher success rate than with ova stimulation. It's a gimmick."

Dr. Virro, who performs GIFT at Markham-Stouffville Hospital, gets starry-eyed when he talks about it. "We try everything else before GIFT, and we are getting women pregnant who couldn't get pregnant any other way."

It's difficult to be a good consumer in an unregulated field, where new treatments or variations on old ones emerge practically monthly and opinions differ drastically on their relative merits. "There should be established protocols for drugs and a maximum number of cycles per patient," says Dr. Virro. "I have patients with tragic histories of infertility, eleven and twelve years, who were run through programs again and again, and it turns out they have blocked tubes, but no one ever bothered to do a laparoscopy."

Any MD can stick up a shingle proclaiming himself (or in relatively rare cases, herself) an infertility specialist. Many patients are too desperate to have a child, or too trusting, or too uninformed, to know what questions to ask or even, given the way the information is presented, how to interpret answers.

By late October, the waiting room had become downright oppressive. Why couldn't appointments be staggered? Would this be happening if the patients were all men? And where were the men — wasn't this their problem too? On two mornings a lone man did slink in with his wife, looking as if he were pretending he'd just come to read the magazines. One day when The Man was absent, a woman tut-tutted, "I feel so sorry for my husband, he's embarrassed about giving the sperm samples, it's very hard for him."

"To hell with the husband!" Emma snapped under her breath. "All they do is ejaculate into a bottle twice a month — *that's* a big deal? Even if part of the problem is his sperm count, it's my body that's supposed to do everything. It's rage at things you have no control over."

By this point, though, she showed more grit than rage. She was positively blasé about the blood tests, and had figured out how to get Dr. Owen's attention: one day, she simply refused to get on the examining table until he answered her questions. "He's not such a bad guy," she decided. And she was following the growth of her follicle with the excitement of a sports fan: "I'm at 1.9 centimetres!"

This cheeriness was in fact somewhat forced. While she was up at 5 a.m., her sister was also awake, nursing a newborn. "I've shut down emotionally because when I think about my sister and her son, there are a lot of overwhelming feelings, anger, that I just can't share, even with Ian," Emma said on day four. Ian was depressed by her seemingly radiant sense of purpose. *Why doesn't she feel as bad as I do?* Their sex life dwindled to abstinence, imposed by emotional distance as well as mathematical calculations. "She was told she might ovulate on Sunday so we stopped two days before that, to store up sperm for good counts," said Ian. By the time it was all over, they hadn't been allowed to have sex for ten days.

After the first insemination, Emma was reflective: "What's hard on men is that they're only involved for two days, and what they see is the worst part of it because they see what, from their perspective, they can't do. Today I looked at Ian's sperm count and said, 'Oh shit, it's poor' — tactful, sensitive wife that I am. I'm thinking, I've gone through all this and you're giving me a lousy sample?! This cycle I've been much stronger, less needy. Maybe that's part of it for Ian: it's bad enough to feel incompetent but then his wife gets to the point where she doesn't share her feelings, so he doesn't even get to provide emotional support. It's becoming totally unconnected to him."

"Primarily my anger is toward life, really, toward God," Ian said separately. "These borderline sperm counts make me feel inadequate. I look at the monitor and think, with a good count would the whole screen be full of those wiggling things?"

After inseminations by both the doctors on call, neither of whom was Dr. Owen, Emma's cheer had evaporated. "The second was the worst. He didn't warm the speculum, just cranked me open, shot the sperm up, rammed the cap in and ran out the door. His only concern was to stay on schedule, and gentle is not the word I'd use to describe his technique," she said, then struggled with her emotions. "I feel I have to justify these doctors to Ian and to you. I don't know why I feel I have to protect them because I have a lot of problems with them myself, but I guess I need to feel that they're somehow nicer or better than they really are because I don't want to really think about the things they do, it's just too upsetting. I'd be in tears all the time."

When November brought no good news, Emma was stunned. *All it takes is one tiny sperm and there were millions. I don't get it.* Ian's anguish was closer to the surface: "I lied when I said disappointment lessens over time. This month I feel absolute despair. I'm not sure how many more times we can do this." In January, they decided to try fertility drugs.

A happy ending. Everyone has a different idea about what that would be. For critics of the NRTs, it would be a redirection of public funds from cure to prevention, massive public education about sexually transmitted diseases, for instance, to try to curb infertility in future generations. Critics as well as supporters of the NRTs focus a lot on the future: future effects, future developments, future applications.

Couples who use the NRTs think of the future somewhat differently: our family, Johnny's first step, Linda's first day of school. Or, no family. Watching our friends have children, then grandchildren, and feeling an ache for the rest of our lives.

There's a peculiar alchemy between reproductive longing and science, which holds out possibilities that continually reinforce desire even when they fail to satisfy it. *We have the technology. I know what's at stake: me, my body, my future.* Who can be blamed for what seems in a certain light to be courage, a leap of faith, even if it's taken in ignorance of just how large the leap might be? And how can we weigh a personal reproductive choice against its possible social consequences?

"To me, it's similar to a hostage situation. If somebody you love is being held hostage, how could you possibly say you wouldn't pay the ransom? You can't in the individual case, because the life of someone you love is at stake," says sociologist Margrit Eichler. "But you could, as a society, before there is a case and something personal is involved, say 'We will not give in to ransom demands, no matter how they come up.' One has to make that distinction, of where one locates the responsibility for these situations arising. And it's wrong to locate it only at the individual level. I understand why people undertake these treatments, but that does not answer the question. Should society as a whole put its resources in that direction?"

For the Dixons there's already been a happy ending. Or maybe it's more of a beginning. "We are closer, we have more or less held the other up and we know much more about what makes the other hurt," says Ian. "If a man and a woman can lie in bed at night and just hold each other and cry or talk in a way that you know absolutely nothing is held back, that I'm glimpsing into her heart at this moment — that can't be bad for you, I don't think. That's what love is supposed to be."

Emma and Ian are still hoping for a baby.

NOTES

1   The U.S. Food and Drug Administration is requiring the makers of pergonal and clomiphene to add information to their labels on the possible link between the drugs and ovarian cancer.
    A review of the database of the Japan Children's Cancer Register from 1985-89 identified significantly more cases of childhood malignant disease in children born to mothers who underwent ovulation induction.

3   In keeping with the recommendations of the Royal Commission, the Ontario government now pays for IVF only in cases of bilateral fallopian tube blockage, and limits payment to three cycles per patient.

18

A PREVENTION ORIENTED APPROACH TO REPRODUCTIVE PROBLEMS: IDENTIFYING ENVIRONMENTAL EFFECTS

Karen Messing & Gail Ouellette

The new reproductive technologies are intended to remedy problems of individual couples. This "curative" approach imposes emotional and financial costs on the couple.[1] An increasing number of groups think it might be more effective to consider a public health approach to these problems, investing in identification and elimination of environmental agents and conditions which may be the source of reproductive problems.

Since the vast majority of women and men of reproductive age are employed, and because of the large number of agents and conditions in the work environment which cause birth defects and hereditary damage (genotoxic and teratogenic agents), one important component of prevention efforts could be to examine the relationship between fertility problems and the working environment.[2] From our own research, complemented by a literature review, we have identified several factors which could affect fertility of women and men.

In order to understand how fertility can be affected by the environment, it is helpful to consider the larger subject of environmental hazards to reproduction. Reproductive problems range along a continuum from total sterility (the inability ever to produce a child) through repeated miscarriages to the inability to produce a healthy child. Exposure to various agents and conditions can produce effects which vary based on the severity of the exposure and the time at which it occurs. For example, sperm can be rendered incapable of fertilizing an egg, the uterus can be made less receptive or the fetus can be damaged. The same agents and conditions which affect one stage may also affect others. For example, exposure to ionizing radiation (such as X-rays or nuclear waste) can damage sperm, eggs and fetuses. If sperm or eggs are severely damaged, pregnancy may become impossible. If fetuses are badly affected, there may be an early miscarriage, so early that the woman is unaware of it. Or the fetus may develop a health problem such as cancer later in life.

Sterility	delayed conception	miscarriage	stillbirth	child with minor health problems	Birth of healthy child

The environment can affect the health of sperm, eggs and fetuses in various ways:

EFFECTS ON MALE FERTILITY.

It has been demonstrated that men's fertility can be affected by various agents found in the workplace and in the environment: heat, radiation, pesticides, metals and pharmaceutical preparations.[3] Smoking can affect sperm concentrations, resulting in a risk not only for smokers but also for workers exposed to high concentrations of smoke (barman, nightclub waiter).[4] Other effects are less well defined. For example, it has been shown that there is lowered fertility among professional drivers,[5] possibly due to the prolonged sitting posture or to vibrations. These agents and conditions may act by damaging genes or by affecting endocrine or sexual functioning. The fact that clinicians often give examination of male functioning second place in their work-ups has slowed efforts to study environmental effects on male fertility.

EFFECTS ON WOMEN'S FERTILITY.

Although books have been written on the effects of the environment on pregnancy,[6] somewhat less is known of the effects on conception. Smoking has been shown to affect women's fertility. In one large study, time to conceive increased in proportion to the numbers of cigarettes the women smoked,[7] and another showed that smokers were more likely to have irregular menstrual cycles.[8]

The work environment has been examined in a few studies. Danish researchers associated infertility problems among women with exposure to noise, metals, dyes, cutting oils, dry cleaning solvents and anesthetic gases.[9] Women's work often involves non-chemical stressors as well, such as a fast workspeed, repetition, lack of control over the work process and lack of respect.[10] Such stressors have physiological effects, which may explain why the same study found lowered fertility among knitting machine operators, cashiers and office workers.

We have studied the effects of women's work on the regularity of the menstrual cycle, a parameter which is related to fertility. We found that exposure of poultry slaughterhouse workers to a variable work schedule and to variable temperatures was associated with an irregular menstrual cycle. Women whose workday began at an irregular time were nearly twice as likely to have irregular cycles or long periods without menstruating (amenorrhea) as those with regular work hours. Those exposed to cold are also about twice as likely to have irregular or missing menses and those exposed to variable temperatures are also twice as likely to have irregular cycles.[8]

ENVIRONMENTAL EFFECTS ON COUPLES

Irregular schedules are increasingly common in Canada, where only 55 percent of parents work from Monday to Friday on fixed schedules between 8 a.m. and 6 p.m.; one may suppose that this is typical of workers of child-bearing age.[11] These irregular schedules may affect fertility both by affecting the ability to conceive (as explained above) or the probability of having sexual relations. How and when a couple makes love may affect the time taken to conceive. This may be affected both by professional working conditions and by the weight of domestic task demands. For example fatigue, tension and general physical well-being may affect one's desire to make love, and travel requirements and domestic work load may affect one's ability to find the time.

OBSTACLES TO RECOGNIZING ENVIRONMENTAL RISKS

Much more energy, attention and money have been expended on finding cures for infertility than on identifying causes. One reason is that infertility has been defined as a medical problem of individuals or couples. The search for collective origins of these problems has been delayed by the individualistic orientation of our health care system. It is not surprising that most studies of environmental effects on the menstrual cycle and on fertility have come from outside North America, from laboratories in Scandinavia or Eastern Europe.

However, we cannot overlook the methodological difficulties which slow research in this area. A major problem in identifying environmental effects on fertility comes from the size of the job. About 100,000 chemicals are in current use and 2,000 new ones are added every year.[12] There is no information about the toxicity of the vast majority of these chemicals, and almost none on the effects of combinations. Only 4 percent of chemicals have even been tested for reproductive toxicity in animal systems.[13]

Testing of other types of workplace conditions lags even further behind. It is more difficult to interest scientists in such "soft" and ill-defined causal factors as schedule compatibility, work postures or exhaustion than it is to induce them to study chemical or physical agents, where conventional methods can be used. Because of the very large number of possible working conditions, and our ignorance of which ones may have important physiological effects, it will be a while before it is possible fully to explore the effects of workplace design and organizational constraints on fertility.

There has been a similar delay in studying psychological effects on fertility. A large variety of working conditions can elicit the "stress reaction," a set of physiological reactions which prepares the body for fight or flight in the face of perceived danger. These reactions involve the parts of the nervous and endocrine systems which control reproduction, and may well affect the capacity to conceive. It has been suggested that stress due to job-related problems may affect fertility.[14]

There has never been a study of the effect of work-related stress on fertility, although the complementary question, the effects of women's hormonal states on their capacity to work, has been extensively explored.[15] It is possible that scientists and granting agencies think it is normal that work be incompatible with reproduction (in the case of women only).

Another problem arises from the tendency of scientists to examine problems in isolation. For example, men's exposure to mercury was related to pregnancy outcome among their wives.[16] However, to study pregnancy outcome requires that pregnancy has occurred and lasted long enough to be detected. But it is also possible that mercury affects the likelihood that conception will occur. It might be advisable to derive statistical techniques which could allow us to consider many possible reproductive problems at once, so as to look at the effects of chemicals on the entire range of function.

Some problems which are presented as methodological, however, are in fact due to anti-worker attitudes on the part of scientists. For many exposures, the only possible source of information has been reports from exposed workers. However, researchers are sometimes reluctant to rely on worker reports, suspecting bias, ignorance or deliberate attempts to exaggerate. (Bias in the choices made by scientists, often with extensive input from employers, on when and what to sample has traditionally aroused less concern.) A growing number of scientists have, however, found that worker exposure reports are reliable, and this obstacle to study is slowly being removed.[17]

THE DESIRE TO PREVENT PROBLEMS

The lack of clear information so far has posed serious problems for prevention strategies. In each workplace, decisions must be taken whether to permit exposure before the final word is in on the exact level of risk. For example, tens of thousands of women worked with video display terminals (VDTs) before the first study of VDT effects on pregnancy. Even now, no one is yet sure whether VDTs pose a danger for pregnancies. In this and many other cases, a decision has been made to place the burden of proof on the worker rather than on the employer. That is, an agent must be proved dangerous before being removed.

In addition, the statistical tests conventionally used exaggerate this burden of proof. In order for scientists to accept the fact that Agent X causes problems for pregnancy, a study must establish the toxic effects with 95 percent certainty.[18] For scientists to be really sure, more than one study must show the same relationship. Given the small numbers of workers in most women's workplaces and the large numbers of potential hazards, it is no wonder that very few dangers for pregnancy or fertility have been established. A decision has been taken to put the burden of proof on the side of minimizing the costs of improvements in hygiene rather than on minimizing questionable exposures.

However, the exposed worker would probably be happier with another standard; it might be better for her/him if scientists suggested taking action even when they had a 50 percent chance of being too cautious rather than a 95 percent chance. But employers and governments are noted for their reluctance to undertake costly clean-ups. Several environmental tragedies have resulted from this sort of delay: the effects of asbestos were officially recognized 60 years after the first insurance companies refused to insure asbestos miners.[19]

Thus, some of the delay in exploring ways to prevent infertility can be attributed to the desire to prevent unnecessary spending. If infertility is to be viewed as a public health problem, society will have to undertake to ensure clean air, better programs to prevent venereal disease, healthy workplaces, improved measures for reconciling workplace and family responsibilities. However, so long as infertility is presented as an individual problem, it is the isolated individuals and couples who are forced to undergo long and painful procedures with limited success. The costs of improving our collective environment must be weighed against the inefficiencies and inconveniences of treating each individual problem separately. Over the long run, it will be cheaper (and of course more humane) to avoid creating fertility problems.

NOTES

1   Conseil du statut de la femme, 1988. *Sortir la maternité du laboratoire,* Gouvernement du Québec.
2   A full treatment of these problems can be found in Messing, K. and Ouellette, G. 1991. *Infertilité et milieu de travail.* Report submitted to the Institut de recherche en santé et en sécurité du travail du Québec. This report was prepared after consultations with Abby Lippman, Louise Vandelac, Louise Guyon, Josée Lafond and Francine Mayer.
3   Wyrobek, A. et al., 1984. "An evaluation of sperm tests as indicators of germ-cell damage in men exposed to chemical and physical agents." *Terato. Carcino. Mutag.* 4: 83-207.
4   Handelsman, D.J., Conway, A.J., Boylan, L.M., Turtle, J.R. 1984. "Testicular function in potential sperm donors: normal ranges and the effects of smoking and varicocele." *Int. J. Androl.* 7:369-82.
5   Sas, M., Szöllos, J. 1979. "Impaired spermiogenesis as a common finding among professional drivers." *Arch. Androl.* 3:57-60.

6   Kenen, Regina, 1993. *Reproductive Hazards in the Workplace*, Haworth Press, New York

7   Howe, G., Westhoff, C. Vessey, M. Yeates, D. 1985. "Effects of age, cigarette smoking, and other factors on fertility: Findings in a large prospective study." *Br Med J Clin Res* 290:1697-1700.

8   Messing, K., Saurel-Cubizolles, M.J., Kaminski, M., Bourgine, M. (1992) "Menstrual cycle characteristics and working conditions in poultry slaughterhouses and canneries." *Scandinavian Journal of Work, Environment and Health* 18:302-309.

9   Rachootin, P. and Olsen, J. 1983, "The risk of infertility and delayed conception associated with exposures in the Danish workplace" *JOM*. 25: p. 394-402.

10 Messing, K. (1991) *Occupational Health and Safety Concerns of Canadian Women*. Ministère du Travail du Canada. Ottawa, Ontario. 110 pages.

11 Lero, Donna S. 1992. "Les régimes de travail des parents et leurs besoins en matière de garde des enfants," *Etude nationale canadienne sur la garde des enfants*. July 1992.

12 Health and Welfare Canada. 1983. "Activities and questions on reproductive health." Ottawa, Canada. *Report of the working group on reproductive health of the Ministry of Health and Welfare*. 145 pp. Since this study was done in 1983, presumably there are now at least 124,000 chemicals in the workplace.

13 Gibbons, A. 1991. "Reproductive toxicity: Regs slow to change." *Science* 254: 25.

14 Wright, J., Allard, M., Lecours, A., Sabourin, S. 1989. "Psychosocial distress and infertility: A review of controlled research." *Int. J. Fertil.* 35:1126-142.

15 For example, Collins, A. 1991. "Premenstrual distress: Implications for women's working capacity and quality of life." In Frankenhauser, M., Lundberg, U., and Chesney, M. *Women Work and Health: Stress and Opportunities*. New York: Plenum.

16 Alcser, K. et coll. 1987. "Occupational mercury exposure and male reproductive health." *Am. J. Ind. Med.* 15:517-529.

17 Joffe, M. 1989. "Male — and female-mediated reproductive effects on occupation: The use of questionnaire methods." *JOM*. 31: 974-979.
    Joffe, M. "Validity of exposure data derived from interviews with workers." *Actes, 23e Congrès international de la médecine du travail*, Montréal. p. 61.

18 These decisions are often made by using "universal" criteria of statistical significance which, in fact, put the burden of proof on the worker and not the exposure. The usual level of significance accepted in epidemiological studies is 0.05. When a risk is accepted at the 0.05 level, this means that the researcher has only one chance in twenty of being wrong in concluding that there is a risk. A study which shows that the researcher would have one chance in ten of being wrong in concluding that there is a risk is considered to be "negative," that is, no risk has been demonstrated. This is true even if the group being studied is so small that there is virtually no chance of demonstrating anything. This point is discussed further in Messing, K. (1991) op. cit. Section 2.

19 Mergler, D. et Desnoyers, L. 1981. "Milieu de travail et santé: Elements d'analyse de la situation québécoise." In Bozzini, L., Renaud, M., Gaucher, D. et Llambias-Wolff, J. *Médecine et société: Les années 80*. Editions St.-Martin, Montréal. pp. 235-248.

19

CHILD SEXUAL ABUSE AND INFERTILITY

Lynda Davies

In the early 1980s I met and worked with Mary, a young woman who was punched or kicked in the abdomen during physical assaults by her husband every month when her menstrual period began.[1] He had wanted her to get pregnant and when she did not, he assaulted her. During the course of my work with her, I learned that she had been sexually abused as a child. The sexual abuse resulted in a sexually transmitted disease, which was not diagnosed until much later. As a result of the sexually transmitted disease, her tubes became blocked and she was infertile. Initially, like many survivors of sexual abuse, Mary believed that she was to blame for the earlier sexual abuse and the current physical abuse. The sexual abuse and the resultant infertility led her to believe that she was damaged and deserved the beatings. Although I had not heard or read about the connections between sexual abuse and infertility, I strongly doubted that Mary was the only woman who had become infertile as a result of being sexually abused as a child. What we learn from women who have been sexually abused is that their experiences are as similar as they are unique. Although awareness of the extent and consequences of child sexual abuse has been growing in Canada for over a decade, infertility as a long-term consequence of child sexual abuse has not yet been explored.

INCIDENCE OF CHILD SEXUAL ABUSE

The resurgence of the women's movement in the 1970s resulted in violence against women and children coming to public attention again.[2] Several journals devoted to violence, including *Child Abuse and Neglect, Victims of Violence, Journal of Interpersonal Violence,* and the *Journal of Family Violence* have recently emerged. There have been numerous and varied reports, conferences and research on child sexual abuse. Provincial governments fund, however inadequately, counselling services for adult survivors of childhood sexual abuse and crisis response teams for children currently being abused. The Canadian Panel on Violence Against Women heard repeatedly about child sexual abuse during its consultation process.[3] The Committee on Sexual Offenses Against Children and Youth (the Badgely Committee) reported extensively on child sexual abuse in 1984. The Committee, mandated to undertake a comprehensive study of the incidence and prevalence of sexual abuse in Canada concluded: "Child sexual abuse is a largely hidden yet pervasive tragedy that has damaged the lives of tens of thousands of Canadian children and youths."[4] Six years later, the Special Advisor on Sexual Abuse to the Minister of Health and Welfare reiterated the concern: "even using a narrow definition of sexual abuse, it is clear that hundreds of thousands of Canadian children have been victims of sexual abuse."[5]

In 1992, the Institute for the Prevention of Child Abuse in Ontario analyzed several large data bases from a variety of sources and found that a conservative estimate of the annual incidence of child sexual abuse involving physical contact in Ontario is 16,500 children, and that the sexual abuse of 5,000 of these children goes undetected.[6]

These studies confirm the experience of feminist counsellors working with recently abused children and with adult survivors of childhood sexual abuse: every year thousands of children in Canada are sexually abused. A significant proportion of child sexual abuse is of the kind which would expose a child to a sexually transmitted disease if the perpetrator of the sexual abuse was infected. Dianna Russell, an American researcher and activist, found that over one quarter of the population of female children have experienced sexual abuse before the age of 14 and well over one third have had such an experience by the age of 18.[7]

Russell also found that, depending on the relationship to the perpetrator, as much as 50 percent of childhood sexual abuse was in the category: "ranging from forced penile-vaginal penetration to attempted fellatio, cunnilingus, analingus, and intercourse — not by force."[8]

The Badgely Committee also found that 50 percent of the most serious forms of sexual abuse (including oral-genital and genital-genital contact) occurred before children were sixteen years old.[9] Both Russell and Badgely have confirmed that children and adolescents are violated in ways which have the potential to expose them to a sexually transmitted disease.

It is now well known that a great deal of sexual abuse of children escapes detection.[10] The consequence of under-reporting is that many children can be infected with STDs and remain asymptomatic, while the damage is being done to their reproductive systems. The Badgely Committee in its population survey found that 84 percent of males and 72 percent of females did not report the abuse to anyone when the abuse was of the kind that includes genital to genital or genital to anal contact. The most common reasons for not reporting were shame and fear of the perpetrator.[11] Russell found that less than 10 percent of abuse was reported to the police.[12] These quantitative data on under-reporting support the experience of survivors and of feminist counsellors who work with adult survivors of childhood sexual abuse. In many cases, the abuse remains unreported until adulthood. When sexual abuse goes unreported, sexually transmitted diseases go undetected and can lead to infertility.

INCIDENCE OF SEXUALLY TRANSMITTED DISEASES IN CHILDREN

Information regarding the true incidence of STDs in children is limited both internationally[13] and in Canada.[14] The Laboratory Centre for Disease Control in Ottawa (LCDC) maintains a data base on the incidence and prevalence of STDs in Canada. Sexually transmitted infections caused by chlamydia trachomatis are the most common.[15]

The information regarding chlamydia infections is only beginning to be available because until 1990 it was not necessary for health care providers in

Canada to report a case of chlamydia to public health authorities.[16] The LCDC cautions that the reported figures are an under-representation of the incidence because under-reporting of STDs is still a major problem. In 1989-90, the number of reported cases of chlamydia in Canada of children 5-14 years was 700, with 80 percent of the children with chlamydia being female.[17]

What these figures tell us is that children are contracting STDs, although the full extent of the problem remains hidden. The reported cases of chlamydia among 15-19 year olds in Canada was 14,736, with 80 percent of the adolescents with chlamydia being female. Some of the adolescents may well have contracted the infection earlier than 15. Clinical studies have found that abuse has occurred for an average of 2-3 years, and in some cases, up to six years prior to the abuse coming to the attention of medical professionals.[18] Any number of adolescents may have been infected at a much younger age as a result of abuse.

Unfortunately, the LCDC figures on chlamydia do not supply information as to how the child or adolescent became infected. The Laboratory Centre for Disease Control notes however that the younger the child, the more likely it is that coercion has taken place.[19] Given the sexual abuse research findings reported earlier and the experience of rape crisis centres in responding to adolescents who have been sexually assaulted, we cannot assume that all adolescents 15-19 years old contracted sexually transmitted diseases as a result of consensual sexual activity.

CHILD SEXUAL ABUSE AND SEXUALLY TRANSMITTED DISEASES.

There is a growing body of knowledge about the actual incidence of STDs in children who are sexually abused. Unfortunately, the majority of Canadian hospitals do not routinely test for sexually transmitted diseases as part of the child sexual abuse protocol.[20] But when routine testing is done at the time of a disclosure of sexual abuse, the clinical findings demonstrate that children are very much at risk of contracting sexually transmitted diseases. Since the early 1980s clinical findings have been reported and their significance discussed in medical journals. A recent Canadian review of this literature found that depending on the population tested, the kind, and duration of the abuse, from 1-17 percent of children and adolescents contract chlamydia as a result of sexual abuse and from 2-20 percent contract gonorrhoea as a result of sexual abuse.[21] The group of children with the highest rate of chlamydia infections were prepubescent girls.[22] The Badgely Committee surveyed eleven hospitals in Canada providing specialized services to children who are sexually abused and found that when testing for STDs was done, 10 percent of children were considered to have an STD as a result of the abuse.[23] As with adults, STDs in children are frequently asymptomatic.[24] A recent clinical study found that 65 percent of children who were diagnosed with chlamydia as a result of sexual abuse did not have any symptoms.[25] While some children and adolescents have no symptoms of a sexually transmitted disease, others have significant symptoms of infection as a result of the sexual abuse. Vaginal, anal and urethral discharges are not uncommon, nor is abdominal pain.[26] Symptoms of disseminated sexually transmitted diseases were found in a group of children 5-13 years of age. Disseminated STDs are those which have moved to and caused infections in other parts of the body. Joint swelling and pain, fever, lethargy and endocarditis were found in these children following sexual abuse and exposure to an STD.[27] The short-term physical consequences are serious enough, but when children have been diagnosed, they can be treated. The thousands of children who do not disclose, are not believed if they disclose, and are not tested even if they are believed, are at risk of becoming infertile as a result of the abuse.

SEXUALLY TRANSMITTED DISEASES AND INFERTILITY

The link between STDs and infertility has been well known for some time.[28] Chlamydia has been called a threat to reproduction and a great problem to public health.[29] Ectopic pregnancies, which frequently result from infections in the fallopian tubes, have been called the new gynaecological epidemic disease.[30] There is growing concern about the long-term consequences of STDs, in particular chlamydia, on fertility. The alarm is based partly on the fact that in many cases infertility can result from silent infections. Silent infections are those that do not create any symptoms for the woman. A child, adolescent or woman can have a silent infection, not know that she has an infection but still become infertile as a result. Silent infections have been found to be a common, if not major cause of tubal factor infertility. In one U.S. study, over 60 percent of women who became infertile had no history of a pelvic inflammatory disease.[31] In another U.S. study, two-thirds of women who had chlamydia infections which resulted in infertility did not know that they had an infection.[32] It has also been recognized in Canada that the long-term effects of sexually transmitted diseases only become apparent decades later when women find themselves infertile.[33] This clinical research on the long-term effects of sexually transmitted diseases on fertility demonstrates that women have become infertile as a result of an unknown infection. We have no way now of knowing how many infertile women have become so as a result of unknown and silent infections which resulted from earlier child sexual abuse.

CHILD SEXUAL ABUSE AND INFERTILITY

The infertility specialists have chosen the image of silent infections to describe what is going on in a woman's body. It is not only the infection that is silent; when it is a result of sexual abuse there is silencing of the abuse itself. For several years the movement to end violence against women and children has sought to break the silence. In the early days of this movement, Susan Brownmiller noted that "sexual offenses against children are barely noticed except in the most violent and sensational instances."[34] In Canada in 1994, there is still a pervasive failure to notice that thousands of children are being abused. No matter how many times the figures are quoted, little happens to alter the social relationships which perpetuate the sexual abuse. No matter how many times women who were sexually abused as children speak out about their experiences, public policy initiatives respond only to the aftermath of sexual abuse, not to the social conditions which perpetuate abuse. The feminist activist, Marie Fortune, has provided an insight as to why the silence has persisted:

Why has the silence persisted? The long and painful history of the patriarchal oppression of women has contributed to denial of sexual violence as a problem. The victims of sexual assault are primarily women and girl children. This victimization of women and girls has been lost in silence, regarded as insignificant. Not coincidentally, this silence has served to maintain the status quo of women's oppression and isolation"[35]

There is a new development which could well function to further silence the sexual abuse of children. Infertility is a social, not a medical problem. As a community, when we strive to find medical and technological solutions to infertility, we move further away from understanding and addressing the causes of infertility. In so doing, we may fail to notice child sexual abuse as a cause of infertility. As technologies are developed that pretend to cure a social problem, we are less likely to work toward eradicating sexual abuse. If we uncritically accept the technologies as a cure for infertility, which they are not, we will be less inclined to challenge the social relations which perpetuate the sexual abuse of children. The new reproductive technologies build on and reinforce those existing social relationships. They do not seek to challenge them.

NOTES

1   Mary is a pseudonym.
2   For a history of earlier movements to end the sexual abuse of children see: Linda Gordon, *Heroes of Their Own Lives: The Politics and History of Family Violence.* Viking, New York 1988; Sheila Jeffreys, *The Spinster and Her Enemies: Feminism and Sexuality 1880-1930.* Pandora Press, London 1985.
3   Canadian Panel on Violence Against Women: *A Progress Report,* Ottawa 1992.
4   Committee on Sexual Offenses Against Children and Youth, *Sexual Offenses Against Children.* Ottawa: Department of Supply and Services 1984. (Hereafter, *The Badgely Report*) Volume 1: 29.
5   Rix Rogers, *Reaching for Solutions: The Report of the Special Advisor to the Minister of National Health And Welfare on Child Sexual Abuse.* Ottawa, Supply and Services 1990, 18.
6   N. Trocme, *Estimating The Scope of Child Sexual Abuse and Neglect in Ontario: A Guide to Understanding Child Maltreatment Statistics.* Research Connection Institute for the Prevention of Child Abuse, Toronto, September 1992, 2-11.
7   Dianna Russell, *Sexual Exploitation: Rape, Child Sexual Abuse and Workplace Harassment.* Sage California, 1984, 194.
8   Dianna Russell, 187.
9   *The Badgely Report.* Volume 1: 179-181.
10 R. Hunter, N. Kilstrom, F. Loda, "Sexually abused children: identifying masked presentations in a medical setting." *Child Abuse and Neglect* 9: 1985, 17-25.
11 *The Badgely Report.* Volume 1:187.
12 Dianna Russell, 194.
13 S. Estreich, G. Forster, "Sexually transmitted diseases in children: introduction," *Genitourin Med 68*: 1992, 2-8.
14 W. Bowie, N. MacDonald, "Management of sexually transmitted diseases in Canada, 1989" *CMAJ* 140: March 1 1989, 499-501.
15 Bowie and MacDonald, "Management of sexually transmitted diseases in Canada"; H. Bryant, "The

Infertility Dilemma: Reproductive Technologies and Prevention" The Canadian Advisory Council on the Status of Women, Ottawa, February 1990

16 *Canadian Diseases Weekly Report* 17:51 December 1991.

17 *Canadian Diseases Weekly Report* 17:51.

18 R. Hunter, N. Kilstrom, F. Loda, "Sexually abused children: Identifying masked presentations in a medical setting"; R. Dube, M. Hebert, "Sexual abuse of children under 12 years of age; A review of 511 cases" *Child Abuse and Neglect* Vol 12, 1988, pp2-8.

19 *Canadian Diseases Weekly Report* 17:51.

20 Dianne Kinnon, and Jo Anne Doherty "Hospital response protocols for child sexual abuse and sexually transmitted disease in children" *Canadian Journal of Public Health.* July-August 1992.

21 D. Lindsay, and J. Embree, "Sexually transmitted diseases: A significant complication of childhood sexual abuse" *Canadian Journal of Infectious Diseases* 3:3 May-June 1992 122-128

22 C. Fuster, and L. Neinsten, "Vaginal chlamydia trachomatis in sexually abused pre-pubescent girls" *Pediatrics* 79:2 235-238.

23 *The Badgely Report,* 2: 740.

24 S. Estreich, G. Forster, "Sexually transmitted diseases in children: Introduction" *Genitourin Med 68:* 1992, 2-8.

25 D. Ingram et al, "Epidemiology of adult sexually transmitted disease agents in children being evaluated for sexual abuse" *The Pediatric Infectious Disease Journal* 11:11 945-950.

26 J. Cupoli and P. Sewell, "One thousand fifty-nine children with a chief complaint of sexual abuse" *Child Abuse and Neglect* 12: 1986 151-162.

27 R. Hunter, N. Kilstrom, F. Loda, "Sexually abused children: Identifying masked presentations in a medical setting," *Child Abuse and Neglect* 9: 1985, 17-25.

28 Heather Bryant, "The infertility dilemma: reproductive technologies and prevention," *The Canadian Advisory Council on The Status of Women,* Ottawa, February 1990; Anne Mullens, *Missed Conceptions: Overcoming Infertility* McGraw Hill, Toronto, 1990.

29 J. Paavonen, and P. Wolner-Hanssen. "Chlamydia trachomatis: A major threat to reproduction" *Human Reproduction* 4:2 1989: 111-124; K. Ramstedt et al, "Risk factors for chlamydia trachomatis infection in 6810 young women attending family planning clinics" *International Journal of STD and AIDS* 3: 117-122.

30 R. Maymon et al, "Ectopic pregnancy, the new gynaecological epidemic diseases: Review of the modern work-up and the nonsurgical treatment option" *Int J Fertility* 37:3 1992: 146-164.

31 R.C. Brunham et al, "Chlamydia trachomatis: its role in infertility" *Journal of Infectious Diseases* 152: 1985, 1275-1282.

32 H. Thejls et al, "Diagnosis and prevalence of persistent chlamydia infection in infertile women: tissue culture, direct antigen detection and serology" *Fertility and Sterility* 55:2 1991, 304-310.

33 W. Bowie, N. MacDonald, "Management of sexually transmitted diseases in Canada, 1989" *CMAJ* 140: March 1, 1989, 499-501.

34 Susan Brownmiller, *Against Our Will: Men, Women and Rape.* Bantam, New York, 1976: 307.

35 Marie Fortune, *Sexual Violence: The Unmentionable Sin.* Pilgrim Press, New York, 1983, xi.

20

THE EVALUATION OF PHARMACEUTICAL PRODUCTS: PROBLEMS OF PHASE IV

Rosanna Baraldi

Diethylstilbestrol, Thalidomide, the Dalkon Shield: these infamous products and medical technologies revealed the possibility of tragic and unexpected consequences for health of untested interventions. More recently, numerous scientific articles have emphasized the considerable risks associated with massive use of ovulation inducers. Where do we stand with regard to the evaluation of the long-term consequences of pharmaceutical products?

In this article, I begin by examining the mechanisms used to evaluate pharmaceutical products in Canada. I then discuss the question of ovulation inducers and illustrate the attitudes of medical researchers concerning the potential long-term effects of these powerful hormonal products.

THE PHARMACEUTICAL INDUSTRY: FORGETTING PHASE IV

The process of marketing a new pharmaceutical product for humans theoretically involves four evaluation phases. In phase I, that is to say, after a new compound has been tested on small animals, the manufacturer asks the Health Protection Branch (HPB)[1] for permission to conduct trials on "healthy volunteers," of whom the number ranges from 20 to 80. During phase II, the drug is tested on 100 to 300 "volunteer patients," i.e., persons having the target disease. In phase III, trials are conducted in hospitals and private clinics on 1000 to 3000 volunteer patients having the target disease. When these phase III trials of the drug's effectiveness are conclusive, the manufacturer files a "new drug submission application" with the Drug Directorate of the Department of Health and Welfare of Canada. The latter examines these applications and may grant authorization to sell (HPB, 1991). It is then that the study of the long-term effects of a product, that "post-marketing surveillance" called phase IV, can begin.[2]

Hence, it is important to realize that the long-term effects of a new pharmaceutical product have not been evaluated at the time of marketing. At best, the product may have been administered to 3000 patients, a limited sample in which even an undesirable reaction with high incidence would have little chance of being noticed (Sneader, 1986). For instance, a retrospective analysis of products withdrawn from the market in recent years showed that several hundred thousand people had to be exposed to the effects of a product before its harmfulness, on the short or medium term, was recognized (Sneader, 1986). If this is true of short- and medium-term effects, we may assume that much more time and the exposure of many more persons are needed before the long-term effects of a product will be identified. We may even assume that a number of long-term effects will remain unknown, given the serious gaps in the application of phase IV.

In Canada, the post-marketing surveillance program relies mainly on voluntary statements from health professionals on the harmful effects of a drug (HPB, 1991) and on the legal obligations of the manufacturer to report all new information on any product having the status of new drug (HPB, 1991) — a new drug is a "pharmaceutical product which has not been sold for sufficient time and in sufficient quantity to establish its harmlessness and its effectiveness when used under the conditions or for the purposes recommended" (HPB, 1991). Clearly, however, the organization of medical work does not favour the observations needed to collect data on the effects of pharmaceutical products, nor do the priorities of the pharmaceutical industry, aimed as they are at the constant development of new products, permit the mechanisms for evaluation to be complete and effective.

With respect to the legal obligations of the manufacturers to report all new information, it is strange, to say the least, that there is no requirement to conduct rigorous, systematic research using controlled studies to evaluate the long-term effects of the products sold. According to a senior official of the HPB post-marketing surveillance program, it is the manufacturer who decides whether or not to conduct studies on long-term effects. However, it is impossible to know what criteria are used by manufacturers in deciding to conduct such research: the Canadian Pharmaceutical Association (CPA) has refused to give us this information or help us to obtain it. In fact, despite repeated, persistent requests for information involving about twenty telephone calls over a period of two months and conversations with more than a dozen people, including three division chiefs at the HPB, we obtained no specific information on phase IV research.[3]

THE AMBIGUOUS ROLE OF THE HEALTH PROTECTION BRANCH: PROTECTION OF THE PUBLIC OR PROMOTION OF THE PHARMACEUTICAL INDUSTRY?

Back in 1985, the Commission of Inquiry on the Pharmaceutical Industry submitted a report which led to the establishment of a series of measures aimed at stimulating the growth of the pharmaceutical industry in Canada (Government of Canada, 1985). Concerning the process of authorization to sell a new product, this report supported the reduction of deadlines for approval and simplification of the modalities of submission of applications by the industry. To our knowledge, a redefinition of phase IV with a view to an effective, rapid evaluation of the long-term effects of pharmaceutical products was not specifically discussed. In connection with the recommendations on the reduction of deadlines, we learn, however, that there is no regulation permitting the HPB to require that manufacturers conduct post-marketing studies, and that a new regulation to this effect would serve to "speed up the approval process [sic]."[4]

Last June, Nicholas Regush pointed out in The Montreal *Gazette* that a series of measures instituted to simplify the process of authorization to sell new products has led to major problems. Thus, reviews of applications from companies have become summary and incomplete, since the deadline of 60 days given to the HPB is clearly inadequate for evaluating and authorizing experiments on human subjects. After this deadline was instituted, only some of the applications submitted by the pharmaceutical industry would end up being examined carefully; the majority got only superficial reviews. In addition, the tendency to replace medical evaluators with other professionals who were not supervised also affected the quality of evaluations. That the HPB frequently has recourse to outside evaluators having connections with or working for the companies concerned, ignoring possibilities for conflict of interest, only compounded the problems (Regush, 1992).

The lack of rigour in the approval process is not without its effects on the evaluation of product quality. To illustrate, let us recall that it took more than twenty years to recognize the significant psychological distress associated with the sleeping pill Halcion, for which the manufacturer apparently did not report all the symptoms observed. And, even when Great Britain banned Halcion in October 1991, Canada simply recommended a reduction in the initial dose (Regush, 1992). As regards Toradol, its classification as a non-narcotic painkiller instead of as a non-steroidal anti-inflammatory, which it is, as the manufacturer admitted last November, not only constitutes a decisive factor influencing when it is prescribed, but also masks consideration of the potentially grave side effects of this type of product (e.g., kidney obstruction and fatal allergic reactions) (Regush, 1992). Similarly, in the case of Imitrex, an anti-migraine medication, it was only seven months after its introduction onto the Canadian market, when cases were reported in Great Britain and Canada, that the manufacturer admitted that this product could affect the coronary arteries of patients with no history of heart disease (Regush, 1992). Lastly, in the case of the Meme implant, it was more than two years after Dr. Pierre Blais, an expert working for the federal government, recommended that the manufacturer Surgitek withdraw its product from the market until its harmlessness could be established that his advice was heeded (Regush, 1991). Though initially ignored, his fears were sufficiently well founded that the breast implant was banned in January 1992, a ban supported in April 1992 by the independent advisory committee on silicone breast implants (Baines et al., 1992).[5]

In the light of these examples, how can we believe that the HPB is really fulfilling its function which, and we quote, is to "protect and improve the well-being of Canadians by determining, evaluating and managing risks to human health" (HPB, 1991). Is it not a conflict of interest to oversee the protection of the public while attempting to stimulate the development of the pharmaceutical industry?

OVULATION INDUCERS: ABUSIVE DISTRIBUTION AND LACK OF EVALUATION

Let us now turn to the case of ovulation inducers[6] which are widely prescribed for women having no ovulation problems (Taymor, 1987; Fishel and Jackson, 1989).[7] The data collected by the World Health Organization (WHO) indicate that ovarian overstimulation syndrome[8] affects 1 to 2 percent of women in whom ovulation is induced and that the frequency of multiple pregnancies in IVF — pregnancies made possible by the use of ovulation inducers — is 25 percent, or 25 times higher than under natural conditions (WHO, 1990; Testart, 1991). We would emphasize that multiple pregnancies lead to a series of complications of which the frequency greatly exceeds that of single pregnancies (see Launslager and Sky chapters). Thus, in IVF babies, perinatal mortality is four times higher, neonatal mortality twice as high and children of very low birth weight (less than 2.5 kg) eleven times higher than in the general population (WHO, 1990; Wagner, 1989).[9]

For several years, some researchers and clinicians have been suggesting that serious long-term consequences could be associated with ovulation inducers. In 1989, an article entitled "Follicular Stimulation for High Tech Pregnancies: Are We Playing it Safe?" reported:

> ... in many patients the plasma oestrogen concentration and the number of ovulating follicles arising in a single stimulated cycle may be equivalent to the product of up to two years of normal ovulation during the natural menstrual cycle. Excessive oestrogen secretion has been implicated in ovarian, endometrial, and breast carcinoma, and excessive gonadotrophin secretion has been implicated in ovarian cancer. Should we be concerned about such exorbitant ovarian stimulation?[10]

The carcinogenic potential of estrogens has been extensively described (Palmund, 1991). Referring to the history of diethylstilbestrol[11] which is an estrogen, Lynch et al. (1990) write:

The administration of estrogen is etiologically linked to cancers of eight organs: breast, cervix, endometrium, ovary, pituitary gland, testicles, kidneys and bone marrow and this has been observed in five animal species: mice, rats, rabbits, hamsters and dogs.[12]

In its 1991 document on human reproductive technologies, the Canadian Medical Association acknowledged the serious problems associated with inducers and emphasized the experimental nature of the medical practices.

... the techniques used in most of these attempts involve a tangible element of risk for women who have recourse to this method. In addition, we sometimes know so little about the long-term effects of these techniques that we might almost say that their use amounts to a stab in the dark... Thus, consent to participation in such interventions can almost mean consenting to unproven techniques.[13]

Despite the numerous criticisms and concerns presented as highly plausible hypotheses, it was not until November 1992, when the Collaborative Ovarian Cancer Group (COCG)[14] published its study in a prestigious American journal, that what we hope will be a "serious" interest on the part of the authorities concerned was first felt. Researchers reported that the risk of ovarian cancer might be three times greater for white women treated with ovulation inducers than for women who did not have fertility problems. Among those who had never been pregnant, the risk of ovarian cancer could be 27 times greater. This was the first study to reveal a statistically significant association between ovulation inducers and ovarian cancer.

Despite the limitations of the data collected, experts with the National Institutes of Health (NIH)[15] consider that the strength of this study lies in the scope of the statistical link — especially among women who did not become pregnant (Spirtas et al., 1993). Describing the COCG results as "provocative" and referring among others to numerous isolated clinical cases reported in American and French medical literature, these experts said it was essential to continue research, keep patients informed, and preserve all medical information and files for the purpose of offering specific information about the nature of this risk (Spirtas et al. 1993).

At the same time, the *Wall Street Journal*, January 14 1993, reported that the U.S. Food and Drug Administration (FDA)[16] was asking manufacturers of ovulation inducers to include information about the risk of ovarian cancer on product labels. A communiqué issued by the FDA estimates that at least 12.5 million prescriptions for these substances had been issued since they first came on the market in the early 1960s.[17] But what about current medical protocols and the health of women on whom these experiments have been carried out for more than 20 years? In 1989, Fishel and Jackson suggested with incredible cynicism:

> ... *if a cause or link between prolonged severe stimulation and ovarian carcinoma were to be confirmed certain patients who have had many years' stimulation treatment could be offered bilateral oophorectomy [ablation of both ovaries] once they were in the menopause.*[18]

In an often obscurely worded 1991 article, the Canadian Medical Association recommended the "evaluation of the scientific validity of various methodologies" before adopting a "public policy on triggering ovulation."[19] In 1993, following the results of the COCG and the unchecked development of human reproductive technologies, concerns were expressed not only about the health of the women for whom inducers are prescribed in the hope of having a child, but also about the health of women who repeatedly "donate ova... without obtaining a reproductive benefit [sic] from this exposure to ovulation inducers."[20]

Through discussion prompted by the COCG results, we learned about an organized and established practice of ova donation in certain American medical centres. In commenting on this practice, Florence Haseltine, Director of the NIH Office of Population Research, declared:

> *There is no excuse for young girls to be getting the drugs to donate eggs .... These are young kids. There's often a $2,000-$3,000 inducement... How do you know their fertility won't be impaired? We're sticking their ovaries with needles (to pirate out the eggs). Will they have early menopause?*[21]

Back in 1647, Dr. W. Harvey already spoke of the risks for the public of collusion between industrial powers and the medical community. He expressed this opinion which still gives pause for reflection today.[22]

> *If we had wanted the college of physicians to do useful work for the population, we should have demanded that they conduct a study on the*

*damage and the benefits of tobacco in general and not a comparative study
of the Virginia plant and that grown in England. But the art of governing
is certainly not the art of protecting citizens as the naive might think.*[23]

CONCLUSION

In the face of the growing number of controversies, sometimes involving
veritable scandals, and given the scope of the uncertainties which have been
barely touched upon here by citing a few cases, it is imperative that phase IV of
the experimental evaluation of pharmaceutical products become a reality and
cease to be a theoretical concept for which neither industry, government bodies
nor the medical community seem to want to assume real responsibility. In the
case of the human reproductive technologies, it is the future health of women
and of children that makes their evaluations essential. The health of the public
— and above all women's health — is otherwise placed at incalculable risk.

ACKNOWLEDGMENT

This work was carried out as part of a research project funded by the CRSH entitled: *Ethics and
Biomedical Experimentation on Humans: Women and Extracorporeal Fertilization.* I wish to thank
Louise Vandelac, research director, for her assistance and our stimulating discussions.

BIBLIOGRAPHY

Baines, J.C., Arseneault, J., Davis, P., Smith, D.C. Rapport sur les prothèses remplies de gel de silicone,
Report prepared for the hon. Benoit Bouchard, Minister Health and Welfare Canada, 1992.

Cabau, Anne. "Dangers des inducteurs de l'ovulation," *La lettre du gynécologue*, 1986, no. 45, pp. 2-4.

The Canadian Medical Association. Les nouvelles techniques de reproduction humaine, Canada, 1991,

Cornel, M.C., Ten Kate, L.P., TeMeerman, G.J. "Ovulation induction, *in vitro* fertilization and neural tube
defects," *The Lancet*, December, 23 1989, p. 1530.

Dieckman, W.J., Davis, M.E., Rynkiewicz, L.M., Pottinger, P.E. "Does the administration of
diethystilbestrol during pregnancy have therapeutic value?" *American Journal of Obstetrics and
Gynecology*, 1953, no. 66, pp. 1063-1075.

Direction générale de la protection de la santé. Les médicaments, la santé et la loi, Ottawa, *Groupe
Communication Canada*, 1991, 76 pages.

Fishel, S., Jackson, P. "Follicular stimulation for high tech pregnancies: Are we playing it safe?," *British
Medical Journal*, 1989, vol. 229, pp. 309-311.

Food and Drug Administration. "FDA asks for fertility drug labeling change," *FDA Talk Paper*, 13 January
1993, 2 pages.

Frydman, R. Fanchin, R., Cornel, C. "Comment contrôler le risque de grossesses multiples et
d'hyperstimulation au cours des simulations ovariennes," *Contraception-Fertilité-Sexualité*, 1992, vol.
20, no.2, pp.223-228.

Goldberg, G.L. et al. "Ovarian carcinoma of low malignant potential, infertility and ovulation induction — Is there a link?," *American Journal of Obstetrics and Gynecology*, March, 1992 pp. 853-854 in Laborie F., "Nouvelles technologies de la reproduction (NTR) risques pour la santé des femmes," unpublished article, 1992.

Gordon, C.V., Wierenga, D.E., "The drug development and approval process" in United States Pharmaceuticals Manufacturers Association, *In Development New Medicines for Women*, 1991

Gouvernement du Canada, Ministère des Approvisionnements et Services Canada, *Rapport de la commission d'enquête sur l'industrie pharmaceutique*, 1985.

Grandjean, H. "La stimulation de l'ovulation comment éviter les grossesses multiples? Le point de vue de l'épidémiologiste sur les résultats," *Contraception — Fertilité — Sexualité*, 1992, vol. 20, no. 2,

Guttfeld, Rose. "FDA says labels of fertility drugs must warn users," *The Wall Street Journal*, January, 14 1993.

Hamburger, J. *Le journal d'Harvey*, Paris, Flammarion, Coll. Folio, 1983.

Herbst, A.L., Ufelder, H., Poskanzer, D.C. "Adenocarcinoma of the vagina: Association of maternal stilbestrol appearance with tumour appearance in young women," *The New England Journal of Medicine*, 1971, no. 284.

Kessler, David A. "Drug promotion and scientific exchange — The role of the clinical investigator," *The New England Journal of Medicine*, 1991, vol.325, no.3.

Klein, Renate and Rowland, Robin. "Women as test-sites for fertility drugs clomiphene citrate and hormonal cocktails," *Reproductive and Genetic Engineering*, 1988, vol. 1, no. 3.

Kulkarni, R., McGarry, J.M. "Follicular stimulation and ovarian cancer," *British Medical Journal*, vol. 299 (6701), 1989.

Lacassagne, A. "Apparition d'adénocarcinomes mammaires chez des souris mâles traitées par une substance oestrogène synthétique," *Comptes rendus biologiques*, 1938, no. 129.

Laborie, Françoise. "D'une banalisation sans évaluation et de ce qui peut s'ensuivre," in J. Testart, *Le magasin des enfants*, Paris, Éditions Francois Bourin, 1990.

Laborie, Françoise (a). "Nouvelles technologies de la reproduction (NTR) risques pour la santé des femmes," Unpublished Article, 1992.

Laborie, Françoise (b). "Nouvelles technologies de la reproduction (NTR) risques pour la santé des enfants," Unpublished Article, 1992.

Lancaster, P.A. "Congenital malformations after *in vitro* fertilization," *The Lancet*, no.2, 1987.

Lynch, H.T. et al. "Diethylstilbestrol, teratogenesis and carcinogenesis medical/legal implications of Its long-term sequelae, including third generation effects," *International Journal of Risk and Safety in Medicine*, 1990, no.1, pp. 171 à 193 in Laborie F., op. cit., 1992 (a)7.

Organisation mondiale de la santé, Bureau régional de l'Europe. Consultation sur la place de la fécondation *in vitro* dans le traitement de l'infécondité — Rapport sommaire, Copenhague, 18-22 June 1990.

Palmund, Ingar. "Risk evaluation and estrogens," *International Journal of Risk and Safety in Medicine*, no. 2, 1991.

Regush, Nicholas. "Health and welfare's national disgrace," *Saturday Night*, April, 1991; "Is Ottawa drug testing bad for our health?," *The Montreal Gazette*, June 6, 1992; "New migraine drug can affect heart, maker concedes," *The Montreal Gazette*, August 31, 1992, pp. A1-A2.

Sneader, Walter. *Drug Development From Laboratory to Clinic*, Great Britain, John Wiley & Sons, 1986.

Spirtas, R., Kaufman, S.C., Alexander, N.J. "Fertility drugs and ovarian cancer: Red alert or red herring?," *Fertility and Sterility*, vol.59, no.2, February, 1993, pp. 291-292.

St-Clair Stephenson, Patricia. "The risks associated with ovulation induction," *Iatrogenics*, 1991, no. 1.

Taymor, M.L. "Use and abuse of clomiphene citrate," *Fertility and Sterility*, vol. 47, no. 2, 1987.

Testart, Jacques et al. *Le magasin des enfants*, Paris, Éditions François Bourin, 1990, 338 pages.

Testart, Jacques. "Introduction," pp. 9-34 in J. Testart, op. cit.

Vandelac, Louise. "L'embryo-économie du vivant... ou du numéraire aux embryons surnuméraires" pp. 117-139 in J. Testart, op. cit.

Wagner, Mardsen G., St-Clair, Patricia A. "Are *in vitro* fertilisation and embryo transfer of benefit to all?," *The Lancet*, October 28, 1989.

Whittemore, AS, Harris, R., Itnyre, J. The collaborative ovarian cancer group. "Characteristics relating to ovarian cancer risk: Collaborative analysis of twelve US case-control studies II. Invasive epithelial ovarian cancer in white women," *American Journal of Epidemiology*, vol. 136, no.10, Nov., 1992.

NOTES

1 The Health Protection Branch will be referred to as the HPB.

2 This information is taken from a recent document prepared in the United States but distributed by the Canadian Pharmaceutical Association (CPA) and accompanied by a letter of presentation from the President, Ms. Judith Erola, who generally endorses the information provided (Gordon and Wierenga, 1991:25).

3 We would mention in passing that the problem of the serious gaps in the application of phase IV is frequently raised in concerned circles. It seems, however, that it is left up to the legal system and the "threat of lawsuits" to establish rules and penalties which would provide an incentive for manufacturers to evaluate the long-term effects of the products sold. Now, if we consider the conservatism of the Canadian legal system in terms of manufacturer responsibility, this legal incentive is far from representing a guarantee.

4 We read: "the Commission recommends that a regulation permit the Health Protection Branch to require manufacturers to conduct post-marketing studies as a condition for the granting of the marketing permit. This provision, which does not exist at present, would enable the Branch to exercise better control over new drugs and speed up the approval process" (Government of Canada, 1985: 412). [Translated from French]

5 In the report submitted to the Minister of Health and Welfare of Canada, the independent advisory committee on silicone breast implants emphasizes the absence of scientific research on the "characteristics, behaviour and effects of these implants" (Baines et al., 1992; 1-recommendations).

6 Gonadotrophins (HMG, HCG, FHS, GnRh) and clomiphene citrate (CC), either alone or combined, are the most commonly used products (Grandjean, 1992: 215-222; Frydman et al., 1992: 223-228; St-Clair, 1991: 7-16).

7 Ovulation inducers are used massively in human reproduction technologies because they permit simultaneous production of several oocytes and the subsequent development of several embryos which will either be transferred to the womb, frozen, donated, destroyed or used in research.

8   The ovarian overstimulation syndrome leads to the formation of ovarian cysts and can endanger the life of an otherwise healthy woman (Cabau, 1986: 3).

9   Although it is known that neurological and sensory anomalies are more frequent in underdeveloped infants, there are no data on long-term morbidity. Likewise, there are no valid data on the number of IVF babies born "healthy," but this number is estimated at 4 to 5 per 100 courses of stimulation (Wagner, 1989: 1928).

10 Fishel and Jackson, 1989: 309.

11 Diethylstilbestrol was the first hormone of the estrogen type synthesized in the laboratory. While its effectiveness and harmlessness had not been established and even though studies on mice had revealed its carcinogenic potential (Lacassagne, 1938: 641) and a control study conducted in 1953 had demonstrated its lack of effectiveness in preventing miscarriages (Dieckman et al., 1953: 1063-1075), this hormone was widely prescribed to pregnant women between 1941 and 1971 in North America and much longer in a large number of other countries. In 1971, the link was established between clear cell adenocarcinoma of young women and exposure to D.E.S. in utero (Herbst et al., 1971: 878-881).

12 F. Laborie, 1992a: 7 [Translated from French].

13 Canadian Medical Association (CMA), 1991: 85 [Translated from French].

14 Whittemore et al., 1992: 1184-1203.

15 Canada's equivalent of the American NIH comes within the mandate of the Department of Health and Welfare.

16 The FDA is the American equivalent of the Health Protection Branch of Health and Welfare Canada.

17 FDA — Talk Paper, "FDA asks for fertility drug labelling change," January 13, 1993.

18 Fishel and Jackson, 1989: 311.

19 AMC, 1991: 88. [Translated from French].

20 Spirtas et al., 1993: 292.

21 Robin Herman, "Fertility Treatment's Long-Term Effects," *Washington Post*, January 12, 1993.

22 By way of example, we would mention that in 1988, sixteen pharmaceutical companies examined by the Senate Committee on Labor and Human Relations in the United States had funded 34,688 medical symposiums at costs exceeding 85.9 million U.S. dollars. In 1974, the same sixteen companies had funded 7519 medical symposiums at a cost of about 6.5 million dollars, calculated taking into account inflation and the value of the dollar in 1988. In the last 17 years, the expenditures incurred by pharmaceutical companies to market drugs to doctors have increased at least thirteen-fold, representing colossal sums of money (Kessler, 1991: 201).

23 J. Hamburger. *Le journal d'Harvey*, Paris, Flammarion, 1983. [Translated from French].

21

THE IATROGENIC EFFECTS OF DES

Harriet Simand

Fifty years ago, a "wonder drug" came on the market. Drug companies in search of profits claimed that it was a safe way to prevent miscarriages. Governments approved the drug despite a lack of proof that it was safe and effective. From 1941 to 1971, hundreds of thousands of Canadian women took their prescriptions of DES (diethylstilbestrol), unwittingly turning themselves and their children into victims of one of modern medicine's biggest blunders.

DES was ineffective in preventing miscarriage but it did have its effects which often did not appear until 20 years later in the children of women who were given DES. These latent effects include cancer, fertility and pregnancy problems in DES daughters and infertility and other reproductive system abnormalities in DES sons. DES mothers didn't escape either. They have a substantially higher risk of developing breast cancer.[1]

Other serious long-term health effects are surfacing as the DES-exposed population ages. The DES-exposed may face an increased risk of developing autoimmune disorders. As DES daughters and sons reach midlife, other potential problems include the possible recurrence of cancer, breast cancer in DES daughters as well as mothers, and increased fertility and prostate problems in men.[2]

There is an unsettling but growing belief that DES is a thing of the past, an unfortunate blemish on the medical horizon. But the DES story is not simply an isolated incident of a "wonder drug" gone horribly wrong. The history, marketing and effects of DES raise complex and disturbing issues such as the efficacy of drug testing, long-term health implications of prescribing drugs to healthy women and the capability and willingness of the medical profession to deal with iatrogenic illness.

DES is an artificial estrogen that was first synthesized in a British laboratory by Sir Charles Dodds in 1938.[3] DES was considered a preferable alternative to natural estrogen because it could be administered orally and produced inexpensively. DES was never patented and consequently, more than three hundred pharmaceutical companies produced DES over a thirty-year period.[4]

In 1939, Eli Lilly and Company (Lilly) and other pharmaceutical companies filed an application with the U.S. Food and Drug Administration (FDA) to have DES approved. The initial request was refused, but the FDA encouraged Lilly and twelve other manufacturers to pool their resources and submit new studies. Lilly chaired this committee and in 1941, the FDA approved DES for use in menopausal women, to prevent lactation, and to treat breast and prostate cancer. Animal research at this time, however, indicated that mice exposed to DES could develop tumors.[5]

DES was approved in 1947 for the prevention of miscarriage based largely on the results of a study performed by researchers at Harvard University involving women who were prescribed DES.[6] Unfortunately, there was no control group consisting of pregnant women who were not prescribed DES, so the results of this study were scientifically questionable.

A double-blind controlled study[7] on the effectiveness of DES by Dr. Dieckmann in 1953 indicated that not only was DES totally ineffective in preventing miscarriage, but that bed rest alone was more effective.[8]

Four years after the Dieckmann study was published in the *American Journal of Obstetrics and Gynecology*, an advertisement for DES appeared in the same journal which stated that DES was "recommended for routine use in ALL pregnancies... bigger and stronger babies too." DES was only contraindicated for use during pregnancy by the FDA in 1971, when it was linked to a rare form of cancer in some of the daughters of women who were prescribed DES.[9]

CURRENT IMPLICATIONS

Infertility is a growing issue in today's society. As a result, medical research is developing a variety of techniques, such as *in vitro* fertilization, to overcome the problem. These discoveries are being hailed as medical breakthroughs but in the light of the DES experience, several issues need to be considered.

Firstly, what are the long-term effects of these treatments? Will any of the hormones presently being used to induce ovulation or assist in embryo transfer, for example, have any long-term effects on the child? The effects of DES appeared twenty years after exposure in utero to the drug. Ill effects from these new treatments may not appear for decades. Yet little caution is being expressed about the possibility of long-term effects. News reports about healthy children being born as a result of the use of new reproductive technologies may be misleading. DES children too appeared normal at birth.[10]

Secondly, the priorities of medical research also need to be examined. While tremendous energy and resources are being channeled into organizing IVF clinics, little time or money is being spent to set up DES screening clinics or to publicize the issue. A greater focus should be placed on identifying and eliminating causes of infertility, rather than simply developing new technological procedures to deal with a problem once it arises.

It is ironic that many DES daughters who are suffering from fertility or pregnancy problems because of DES, are now the ones undergoing new infertility treatments. New technology is being touted as the solution to problems created by previous technological mistakes.

Finally, the DES issue has demonstrated that compensation for the DES-exposed has proven difficult to obtain in Canada. As of 1993, there have been no DES lawsuits in Canada although several have been successful in the U.S.A. We must ensure that redress is more accessible for victims of ill-tested drugs, that proper compensation is provided to those affected, and companies must be forced to provide safer, well-tested treatments.

However, we should not be concerned solely with future compensation for victims of other technological errors. Rather, we are faced with rethinking our approach to issues like DES, remembering that caution and prevention are always our first and best options. We should focus more on preventing these tragedies from arising instead of expecting legal or medical solutions once the damage has occurred.

Among the best vehicles for public education on these issues are grassroots organizations such as DES Action Canada. When people organize and educate themselves, they become best able to identify and confront issues that would otherwise become lost in the workings of larger institutions.

DES is a tragic part of medical history, but it is also the present for the DES-exposed who live every day watching and waiting for symptoms. They are living proof that the iatrogenic effects of treatments and technologies must be considered in the long-term and that the transgenerational aspect of any new reproductive technology must receive serious consideration.

The DES story is also the future. We all stand to gain from the light that appropriate future research will shed on similar problems.

NOTES

1   R. J. Stillman, "In utero exposure to diethylstilbestrol: Adverse effects on the reproductive tract and Reproductive Performance in Male and Female Offspring," *American Journal of Obstetrics and Gynecology* 142 (1982), pp.905-921.

2   Jane E. Brody, "Adult years brings new afflictions for DES 'babies'," *The New York Times* , February 10, 1993.

3   Joyce Bichler, *DES Daughter,* New York: Avon Books, 1981, p. 187.

4   Abel v. Eli Lilly & Co., 289 N.W. 2d 20 (Mich. CT App. 1979).

5   A. Lacassagne, "Apparation d'adenocarcinomes mammaires chez des souris mailes traitées par un substance oestrogene synthetique," *Compte Rendus Biologiques* 129 (1938), p. 641.

6   O.W. Smith, "Diethylstilbestrol in the prevention and treatment of complications in pregnancy," *American Journal of Obstetrics and Gynecology* 56 (1948), pp.821-834.

7   This is a study where neither the subjects nor the researchers know who is receiving the experimental drugs or the placebo.

8   W. J. Dieckmann et al., "Does the administration of diethylstilbestrol during pregnancy have therapeutic value?" *American Journal of Obstetrics and Gynecology* 66 (1953), pp. 1062-1081.

9   A. Herbst et al., "Adenocarcinoma of the vagina: Association of maternal stilbestrol therapy with tumor appearance in young women," *New England Journal of Medicine* 284, (1971), pp.878-881.

10 Anita Direcks, "Has the DES lesson been learned?" *DES Action Voice* 28 (Spring 1986) pp.1-2.

22

PROCREATION AND THE CREATION OF MEANING: STUDYING THE NEW REPRODUCTIVE TECHNOLOGIES

Maggie MacDonald

What are the new reproductive technologies? Doctors promote them as therapeutic treatment for infertility; infertile couples hold to them as hope for genetically linked children; pro-life groups reject them as tampering with nature; and feminists submit that they are yet another example of the patriarchal appropriation of reproduction. In short, they are the subject of intense debate arising from contested meanings of biological reproduction and kinship that are culturally, socially, and historically constructed.

What, then, is the meaning of reproduction that allows for the development of the new reproductive technologies in Canada? And what are the implications of such a meaning for women? To address these questions I examine metaphors for procreation that appear in the briefs to the Royal Commission on New Reproductive Technologies. Metaphors allow procreation to be discussed through symbolic associations with other things, thus, they imply culturally specific attitudes, behaviours, and power relations (Sapir and Crocker, 1977). Women understand their bodies not only phenomenologically, but according to dominant cultural representations. Metaphors for procreation are thus part of a powerful cultural order that informs women's self-perceptions and conditions us to behave in certain normative ways, whether we are mothers or not (Graham, 1976; Martin, 1987). Metaphors found in the briefs from the Royal Commission reveal a cultural construction of procreation which has the effect of limiting women's sexual and procreative roles according to the system of patriarchy.

I examine four metaphors for procreation as used and evaluated by the four main groups involved in the Royal Commission debate: Medical Groups and Individuals, Pro-Life/Christian Groups, Women's Groups, and Infertile Groups and Individuals. I discuss the implications of each metaphor for women, and explore strategies for women to move past the reproductive reality and gendered identity that these metaphors construct (Daly, 1978).

THE NATURAL ORDER

This metaphor characterizes procreation as part of an underlying force that directs and controls the entire world, alternately known as the laws of Nature, or simply as Nature. Historically flexible interpretations of the concept — from biological, to normal, to moral, to drug-free — allow it to be manipulated towards a variety of ends.

The *natural order* metaphor, present in virtually all Pro-Life/Christian Groups briefs, is constructed out of organic imagery to evoke a model of procreation as part of a human ecosystem; like a tree bears fruit, humans beings bear children. It dictates a moral order in which: the patriarchal family is "the basic cell of society" (Pro-Life/Christian 4); procreation occurs exclusively within the "the organic web of marriage and family" (Pro-Life/Christian 5); and children are "the fruit of marriage" (Pro-Life/Christian 3).

To a far lesser extent, Medical Groups use the *natural order* to assert that reproduction is a basic physiological function, one of the "basic drives of human kind" (Medical 2). Infertile Individuals also assert that "one of the basic human needs is the need to reproduce" (Infertile 4) to legitimate the desire for children as natural. For both groups, infertility is seen as an inversion of the *natural order* — a disease, a natural disaster.

Negative consequences for women of viewing procreation as part of the *natural order* arise from the essentialist arguments that this metaphor puts forth: that a real family includes genetically linked children, that fatherhood is defined by genetic paternity, that a real woman naturally desires children. First, the presumed naturalness of the patriarchal family means that infertility is considered to be a legitimate problem for married heterosexual couples only. Furthermore, it reflects a concern for maintaining an evaluation of genetic paternity as the real "act of creation" and as the most important social/legal relationship (Rothman, 1989). The focus on genetic paternity also legitimates doctors' use of NRTs to restore the *natural order*, often with painful consequences:

> *The infertile couple can no longer merely accept their infertility as a sort of mysterious incapacity inflicted by fate; instead they must resort to lengthy, expensive, painful, and exhausting diagnostic and surgical procedures. if they fail to make full use of all that medicine offers them, then they seem to have willfully chosen their infertility (Overall, 1987:253).*

The prescription of maternal nurture in the patriarchal family, Pfeffer and Wollet (1983) suggest, continues to allow infertility to undermine the core of the identity of many women. Maternal nurture is problematic in the other direction as well, in that it creates tension between women's actual experience of procreation and the ideals of women as selfless and altruistic (Oakley, 1986, Ginsburg and Tsing, 1990, Raymond, 1991).

Women's Groups, nevertheless, use a version of the *natural order* to some positive ends. To articulate opposition to NRTs, one group asserts that "NRTs intervene into the human body — women's bodies, children's bodies — in much the same way we have intervened into the ecosystem of our planet" (Women's 1). The women's health movement has effectively used this metaphor to regain some control over procreation, as the recent legalization of midwifery in Ontario demonstrates. However, Reissman (1983) argues that part of the agenda of the natural birth movement has simply been co-opted by the medical establishment and turned into a another consumer choice focused on issues like pharmaceutical pain management and location of birth while larger issues of control are silenced.

SUPERNATURAL CREATION

This metaphor for procreation characterizes the life of a child as having been given or created by a divine, disembodied higher being. The predictable use of this metaphor by Pro-Life/Christian Groups overlays the *natural order* metaphor for procreation constructing a model of procreation as naturally supernatural. Children are "created by a creator who has ultimate power and authority over his creation" (Pro-Life/Christian 1). Medical Groups too, use a version of this metaphor which claims for medical doctors the power to give life. "We have engendered," one doctor writes, "two sets of quadruplets, two sets of quintuplets" (Medical 6). Through technology, doctors make their work appear analogous or even superior to acts of *creation* usually reserved for God. One doctor states, "I would simply feel that if a god cannot accommodate the needs of couples to bear children then he or she is a poor god" (Medical 2).

Infertile People also employ the *supernatural creation* metaphor for procreation. To them children are a miracle, something made possible through IVF. "IVF is a miracle or at least the possibility of a miracle" (Infertile 3), one woman writes. "I live the wonderful reality of parenting a child brought to life by IVF" (Infertile 1), writes another.

These versions of the *supernatural* model of procreation are problematic in that women appear as vessels for the creative acts of others, but are excluded themselves from the power to give life (Delaney, 1992; Weigle, 1989). Indeed, the Pro-Life/Christian Group's overlay of *supernatural creation* on the *natural order* specifies the creative, life-giving elements as masculine. The medical version facilitates a neat transfer of generative power from God to doctors via medical technology. Consequently, women's acts of bodily procreation are ignored or devalued — limiting our self-worth and social worth and justifying the regulation and control of women's sexuality and procreation.

Some Women's Groups do, however, refer to a *supernatural* element in procreation in which the power resides within women themselves. It is "women who create and gestate" (Women's 4), one group writes. Conception is "a woman's power" (Women's 11), writes another. An embodied, empowering version of *supernatural creation*, this metaphor does not feature women as vessels for the creative acts of others but as creators themselves.

THE (RE)PRODUCTION LINE

In this metaphor the human body is seen as an assemblage of machines on an industrial production line, making babies for the consumer market. The *(re)production line* encompasses several "embedded metaphors" (Lakoff and Johnson, 1980) including: the *body as a machine,* in which women's bodies are seen as machines, made up of functioning parts in a system, governed by a "biological clock"; *body parts as raw materials,* including ovum, sperm and uterus; *procreation as work,* in which the carrying and bearing of children is exclusively female work; *doctors as managers,* in which labour management and quality control are provided by obstetricians, gynaecologists and fertility specialists; and finally; the *child as a product.* Infertility by this model is a breakdown, a failure of the machine to produce, due to a defect in the machinery, raw materials or labour force. Significantly, the *(re)production line* is also a consumer model, incorporating concepts of private ownership of body parts, remuneration for procreative labour and legal ownership of children. Dialogues of reproductive choice and parenting options illustrate this aspect of the metaphor. If the expressions of the *(re)production line* metaphor seem banal it is because they are the conventional way of talking about fertility, pregnancy, and childbirth in our society. Yet the term reproduction is itself an industrial metaphor — first introduced at the end of the 18th century (Delaney, 1991).

Medical Groups use this metaphor extensively, illustrated by metonymical references to "pregnancy rates" (Medical 6), "success rates in producing a term infant" (Medical 7), "uterine environments" (Medical 4) and "reproductive outcomes" (Medical 1), which invoke the image of the *(re)production line.* Infertile individuals also use the *(re)production line* metaphor for procreation. "I was almost thirty-five and the biological clock was ticking away steadily" (Infertile 6), wrote one woman. They appeal to *doctors as managers* of their fertility to the extent that one woman remarked, "I was beginning to feel that somehow my body was incapable of functioning without the help of a specialist" (Infertile 5). Equally prevalent in this set of briefs is the *child as a product* metaphor depicted by the dialogue of parenting options, choices and goals. Express preference for "children that are genetically our own" (Infertile 2) is unanimously given.

Given the feminist analysis of procreation, one would expect that briefs from Women's Groups would eschew the *(re)production line* metaphor for procreation. Instead, they deliberately rework it to one in which "women own their own reproductive processes" (Women's 6). As owners/managers/labourers women embrace the privatized, commodified *(re)production line* through the dialogue of "reproductive choice" and "parenting options," including such ubiquitous terms as "birth control," "planned parenthood" and "selective abortion." Reformulated as a woman-owned *(re)production line* , the metaphor shows that we have come to see fertility as something we control — a kind of feminist vision of liberation through widespread access to abortion, contraception and reproductive technologies (Firestone, 1970; DeBeauvoir, 1976 (1952)). However, it is still highly questionable how much personal reproductive choice women actually exercise (Hynes, 1991). Although the woman-owned *(re)production line* wishfully omits *doctors as managers,* it is medicine, along with the state, that ultimately define the character and control the direction of medical technology; access to reproductive technology demonstrates traditional family norms, reinforces male and female roles (Stanworth, 1987), and reinforces class and race hierarchies (Corea, 1985). Overall says that reproductive technology has "a paradoxical effect on reproductive freedom" (1989) and may actually serve to reduce women's choices. In particular, she suggests that fetal sex pre-selection will allow people to act on biases against female babies, promoting further exaggeration of existing sex roles.

This metaphor is problematic for women in other ways as well. Because the *(re)production line* breaks the body down into parts, women are separated not only from their bodies but also from their labour. "Scrutiny of the internal female organs has led to greater medical control of women's bodies, and scrutiny of birthing and labour has led to the same result" (Martin, 1990: 302). Women are fragmented individually and as a group, discouraging resistance, while the myth of choices deflects attention from very real social relations of dominance involved in procreation (Corea, 1985; Martin, 1987).

In addition, the machine/labour/owner of the factory, is still judged in terms of parts, performance and product. Obstetrical "risk factor ideology" (Quéniart, 1992:161) embedded in the *(re)production line* focuses emotional blame on women for flawed parts, performance or products and even suggests legal liability for the condition of fetuses (Overall, 1989). Prenatal screening and fetal surgery, for example, enable us to make increasingly detailed specifications about the "type" of child we want — increasing society's abhorrence of deviance and a tendency towards commodification (Overall, 1987).

Furthermore, the woman-owned *(re)production line* does not propose an alternative to infertility as a breakdown, an inability of the machine to produce. Women continue to bear the responsibility for infertility and even for "failed attempts at IVF" (Women's 1). Ultimately, the *(re)production line* transforms the social relations of procreation into property relations (O'Brien, 1981), thus limiting social and emotional aspects.

THE FETUS AS AN ASTRONAUT

From the increasingly medicalized process of pregnancy and birth emerges the image of the "fetus as an astronaut-in-the-uterine-spaceship" in which the embryo/fetus is imagined as a fully human person/patient, distinct from its mother, captain of the vessel, controlling its own destiny and exploiting the natural resources of its mother's body (Daly, 1978:58).

Medical briefs commonly assert that "the fetus may be properly regarded as a patient" (Medical 4), or "the fetus [is] a candidate for intrauterine therapy" (Medical 3). Pro-Life/ Christian briefs lay the ground for the *fetus as an astronaut* metaphor when they claim that it is "an undeniable scientific fact that a new, genetically unique, and complete human life begins at the moment of conception" (Pro-Life/Christian 2). Ubiquitous use of the terms "unborn child," "unborn person," "pre-born human person," refer to a more detailed characterization:

> The preborn child is separate and distinct from its mother. The child develops his own space capsule (the amniotic sac), his own life line (the umbilical cord), and his own root system (the placenta). These all belong to him, not to the mother... The preborn child enlarges its mother's breasts, softens her pelvic bones and determines his/her own birthday (Pro-Life/Christian 6).

Viewing the fetus as a person/patient both facilitates the anti-abortion rhetoric of the Pro-Life/Christian briefs, and is advantageous to the medical agenda as well. By imagining the fetus as a tiny potential patient, more patients are created for doctors to treat — patients that are more interesting, more expensive, more experimental, patients that require specialists.

More importantly, the metaphor raises the issue of who is to control the captain of the vessel, the new person/patient. Husbands, doctors, and increasingly, the state (Daly, 1978:58), by claiming to represent the best interests of the fetus, justify control over women's sexuality, pregnancy and birth and even suggest legal liability (Overall, 1987). Medically and legally speaking, women are increasingly seen in an adversarial relationship to the fetus. Overall cautions:

The possibility exists that proposals to require certain restrictions on the mother's behaviour, in the interest of allegedly protecting fetal life and well being, could be the result of the growing technological focus on the fetus (Overall 1987:250).

As more attention is drawn to the fetus, the pregnant or birthing woman is increasingly eclipsed (Rothman, 1986; Stanworth, 1987). This metaphor encourages a view of women as containers, and fails to see pregnancy as a whole. This may contribute to the feelings of alienation many women talk about in their pregnancy and birthing experiences (Quéniart, 1992). Ultimately, the *fetus as astronaut* metaphor features women in positions of lack of control. It supports medical and legal control over women's bodies and their children, detracts from the freedom of pregnant women, and is continuous with a version of patriarchy that emphasizes social and legal control of sexuality and procreation by men. This metaphor is utterly absent in the Women's Groups, one of which asserts that "the fetus is not an entity unto itself but is wholly and entirely reliant upon the will of the woman in whose body it is developing" (Women's 4).

CONCLUSION

Current conventional metaphors for procreation that appear in the briefs to the Royal Commission on NRTs in Canada are seriously problematic for women, linked as they are to patriarchal definitions of women and children as property, facilitated by the religious presumption of the naturalness of the patriarchal family and by conventional medical definitions of the body as a machine. The invisibility of women's experience is symptomatic of every model for procreation, from the conservative *natural order* to the radical *fetus as an astronaut*. Women are chosen to disappear, regardless of the model, reducing the potential for a kind of group consciousness among women required for social change (O'Brien, 1981).

Attempts to participate in the dominant symbolic order by Women's Groups and Infertile Individuals are limited politically. It may be that women use symbolic images for procreation "in the language of men" because the social organization of certain experience, and hence our way of talking about it, is divorced from "lived actuality" in its need to conform to certain bureaucratic and scientific ways of recording and understanding. (Spender, 1980; Kirby and McKenna, 1989; Smith, 1990)

Yet several examples in the briefs of Women's Groups and Infertile Individuals defy this grim analysis and demonstrate instead that women are capable of shifting back and forth between dominant "outsider" knowledge and authentic "insider" knowledge (McCormack, 1989). Furthermore, the way in which women are both able to participate in and transcend the dominant symbolic order of procreation, points towards viable political strategies.

Some scholars suggest that positive images and metaphors for conception, pregnancy and birth can be generated and disseminated by women's participation in formerly restricted discourses such as medicine (Wearing, 1984; Martin, 1987). Tomm, however, rejects participating in *(re)production line*-like metaphors in favour of models that cannot be owned, bought or sold. She suggests that women, in order to "transcend patriarchal knowledge," have to have new images that come from their own experience (1992:209). Below I explore several examples from the briefs that are both participatory and transcendent.

A variation on *supernatural creation* that I have already touched upon, is the image of women as creators. Part metaphor, part embodied reality, the statement that it is "women who create and gestate" (Women's 4) incorporates both spiritual and bodily elements and seems to acknowledge women's willful action in procreation. Another positive alternative is a model of pregnancy expressed as a unity, as "an interplay of physiological, psychological, and sociological being" (Women's 8) instead of as a mark of natural, inevitable vulnerability. Several intervenors develop the maternal infant relationship into a model for society: the "mother/child unit is the smallest family unit... the very cornerstone on which our society is built" (Women's 7). Not confined to the patriarchal family, it confirms women's centrality in procreation. And because it leaves room to "accept and value the various kinds of family — two parent, single parent, childless, lesbian, extended, or close friends" (Women's 5), it does not necessitate the invisibility and/or punishment of mothers in non-traditional families.

The image of women as caretakers or gardeners of human life also appears in the Women's Groups briefs. Though hardly a blueprint for women's emancipation, the suggestion that to "be a parent, to be the nurturer of another human life is not a right, it is a responsibility" (Women's 10) presents a code for personal and societal relationships profoundly different from, and more palatable than, parenthood as a consumer option.

Ultimately, some of the most plainly powerful passages in the briefs are non-metaphoric, as is the following summary of hospital birth:

> We are anethesized [sic], our bellies are cut, our perineums are cut (the skin between the vagina and the rectum)... our legs in the air while large metal forceps are inserted into our vaginas to pull babies out. We have needles and tubes going in and out of our bodies. We are bruised and we bleed (Women's 7).

Not mystified, nor obscured, nor politicized by metaphor, this passage helps us to see what is really happening. It also helps us to see how conventional metaphors shape our experience and gloss the unspeakable. One of the keys to transcending oppressive metaphors for procreation is to make clear the process by which they rule us (Benston, 1989) — and phenomenological descriptions can do that. Non-technical, non-metaphoric language can also reduce the gap between lay and expert knowledge — another key strategy for women wanting to understand and control their own reproductive selves, and to act in their own best interests. When infertile women speak about themselves without metaphor as in the statement "I am infertile" (Infertile 2), or in saying "laparoscopy results revealed that my left tube was scarred badly and my right tube was not as scarred and open" (Infertile 6), the layers of negative value are reduced from infertility — the guilt, the shame, the loss of control.

Another alternative to the pathology model of infertility is the view fostered by some intervenors in the Women's Health group of "infertility as a symptom of unbalance" (Women's 3), in need of support not fixing. Terms such as "fertility enhancement" (Women's 2, Women's 9) replace therapy and treatment, eliminating harsher images of the broken-down body.

Though not universally applicable to all women and all procreative experience, these alternatives include and express a diversity of women's "lived actualities." And to greater or lesser extents, they share some common themes: they restore women to the central place in procreation; they reintegrate and reassemble women's bodies and the mother/infant unit; and they put them both back in emotional and social space. Clearly, women are not confined to the dominant symbolic order and by resisting, women's own models for procreation can translate into action. For example, Martin (1987) found that by concealing or delaying announcement of the fact that they were in labour, women in her research group actively subvert the medical model of labour and birth as a timed and monitored production, relying instead on their own authoritative models.

In summary, the meaning of reproduction does not remain static over time but rather is part of a "dialectical process which changes historically" (O'Brien, 1981:21). As reproductive technology emerges as a powerful force influencing this dialectic, I have taken the opportunity to examine both constant and (re)emerging symbolic themes — including some more emotionally positive and politically viable alternatives for reproduction offered by women themselves. For when women's procreative experiences are studied, new stories come to light that can change our social and historical understanding and can ultimately change society (Miles, 1985).

BRIEFS CITED

MEDICAL GROUPS AND INDIVIDUALS

1 Fertility Clinic, Chedoke/McMaster Hospitals
2 Department of Obstetrics and Gynaecology, University of Alberta
3 Society of Obstetricians and Gynaecologists of Canada — Genetics Committee
4 Dr. Philip R. Wyatt, Clinical Genetics Diagnostic Centre, North York General Hospital
5 Department of Obstetrics and Gynaecology, University of Western Ontario

6   Dr. Perry Phillips, IVF Canada
7   Dr. Patrick Hewlett, Gynaecologist, Women's College Hospital

PRO-LIFE/CHRISTIAN GROUPS

1   Canadian Baptist Federation
2   Fort Smith Pro-Life Group
3   Roman Catholic Diocese of Saskatoon
4   Friends of the Family
5   Family Forum
6   Right to Life Association of Toronto and Area

WOMEN'S GROUPS

1   National Action Committee on the Status of Women
2   Women's Health Clinic
3   Fertility Management Services Edmonton
4   The Coalition for Reproductive Choice
5   Women's Health Interaction
6   Canadian Research Institute for the Advancement of Women
7   The Maternal Health Society
8   South Surrey/White Rock Women's Place
9   Peterborough Women's Health Care Centre
10 Planned Parenthood Toronto
11 Dawn: Disabled Women's Network Toronto

INFERTILE GROUPS AND INDIVIDUALS

1   Individual Woman
2   Couple
3   Couple
4   Vancouver Infertility Support Group
5   Couple
6   Couple

BIBLIOGRAPHY

Benston, Margaret Lowe. "Feminism and system design: questions of control." in Winnie Tomm (ed.). *The Effects of Feminist Approaches on Research Methodologies*. Waterloo: Wilfred Laurier University Press 1989.

Corea, Gena. *The Mother Machine*. New York: Harper and Row 1985.

Daly, Mary. *Gyn/Ecology*. Boston: Beacon Press 1978.

De Beauvoir, Simone. *The Second Sex*. New York: Knopf 1952.

Delaney, Carol. *The Seed and The Soil*. Berkeley: University of California Press 1991.

Firestone, Shulamith. *The Dialectic of Sex*. London: Paladin 1972.

Ginsburg, Faye and Anna L. Tsing (eds.). *Uncertain Terms*. Boston: Beacon Press 1990.

Graham, Hilary. "The social image of pregnancy: Pregnancy as spirit possession" in The *Sociological Review*. 24(2) pp.291-308 1976.

Hynes, Patricia. (ed.). *Reconstructing Babylon*. Amherst: Amherst Institute of Women and Technology 1991.

Kirby, Sandra and Kate McKenna. *Experience Research Social Change: Methods from the Margins*. Toronto: Garamond Press 1989.

Lakoff, George, and Mark Johnson. *Metaphors We Live By*. Chicago: University of Chicago Press 1980.

MacCormack, Thelma. "Feminism and the new crisis in methodology" in Winnie Tomm, (ed.). *The Effects of Feminist Approaches on Research Methodologies*. Waterloo: WLU Press 1989.

Martin, Emily. *The Woman in the Body*. Boston: Beacon Press 1987.
"The ideology of reproduction and the reproduction of ideology" in Faye Ginsburg and Anna L. Tsing (eds.) *Uncertain Terms*. Boston: Beacon Press 1990.

Miles, Margaret. (ed.). 1985. *Immaculate and Powerful: The Female in Sacred Image*. Boston: Beacon Press 1989.

Oakley, Ann. *The Captured Womb: A History of the Medical Care of Pregnant Women*. Oxford: Basil Blackwell 1986.

O'Brien, Mary. *The Politics of Reproduction*. London: Routledge and Kegan Paul 1981.

Overall, Christine. "Reproductive technology and the future of the family" in Greta Hofman Nemiroff (ed.) *Women and Men*. Toronto: Fitzhenry and Whiteside 1987.

— (ed.) *The Future of Human Reproduction*. Toronto: The Women's Press 1989.

Pfeffer, Naomi, and Anne Woollet. *The Experience of Infertility*. London: Virago 1983.

Quéniart, Anne. "Risky business: medical definitions of pregnancy" in Dawn Currie and Valerie Raoul, (eds.). *The Anatomy of Gender*. Ottawa: Carleton University Press 1992.

Raymond, Janice G. "Of eggs, altruism and embryos" in Patricia Hynes (ed). *Reconstructing Babylon*. Amherst: Amherst Institute of Women and Technology 1991.

Reissman, Catherine Kohler. "Women and medicalisation: A new perspective" in *Social Policy*. (14) pp 3-18 1983.

Rothman, Barbara Katz. *Recreating Motherhood*. New York: WW Norton 1989.
The Tentative Pregnancy. New York: Viking 1986.

Sapir, J. David and J. Christopher Crocker. *The Social Use of Metaphor*. Philadelphia: University of Pennsylvania Press 1977.

Smith, Dorothy. *The Conceptual Practices of Power*. Toronto: University of Toronto Press 1990.

Spender, Dale. *Manmade Language*. London: Routledge and Kegan Paul 1980.

Stanworth, Michelle, (ed.) *Reproductive Technology: Gender, Motherhood, and Medicine*. Cambridge: Polity Press 1987.

Tomm, Winnie. "Knowing ourselves as women" in Dawn Currie and Valerie Raoul, (eds.). *The Anatomy of Gender*. Ottawa: Carleton University Press 1992.

Wearing, Betsy. *Ideologies of Motherhood*. Sydney: Allen and Unwin 1984.

Weigle, Marta. *Creation and Procreation*. Philadelphia: University of Pennsylvania Press 1989.

23

THE INDUSTRIALIZATION OF LIFE

Louise Vandelac (translation by Sheila Fischman)

Is there anyone who has not been stunned to read a headline like "Pregnant with 12 Babies?"[1] Or been startled by "Spare Twin in the Freezer," "Fetus Farming Could Become Reality in Canada" or "Granny Gives Birth to Her Own Grandsons?"

What about egg donation to create pregnancies at age 50, 60 or even 62? Or preconception agreements that provide for transferring embryos to the wombs of two, three, or four women at the same time, who will then turn over the three, four, or five infants they bear to the contracting couple? (See also Eichler and Sherwin.) What about the tens of thousands of frozen embryos around the world patiently waiting in sky-blue nitrogen until they too are used for gestation, donation or research? Or the work on an artificial uterus being done in laboratories at Canadian livestock breeding centres, already the leading exporters of cattle clones? What will be the future of sex selection techniques that have already created a deficit of several million women around the world?

Into what brave new world are we being ushered by reproductive technology and the new techniques in genetics? Our most fundamental reference points have already been shattered: our notions of life, death, mother, father, time, identity and sexual difference, central to our understanding of and relationship to human diversity, are irrevocably altered.

Whatever else can be said about them, these new developments, unthinkable only yesterday, are becoming more and more commonplace with every passing newspaper article, with every passing day. It sometimes seems as if our day-to-day experience has taken us well beyond such fictional creations as Faust or Frankenstein, or even the most astonishing predictions of Aldous Huxley. Indeed, it has reached the point where some people, confusing fact with fiction, wonder if "test tube babies" really are born in test tubes, while others think of "male pregnancy" as virtually a *fait accompli*, unaware that the media madness on the subject was a hoax perpetrated by an Australian newspaper.

How can we separate dream from reality when one of my students, out on her bicycle, is accosted by a couple in a car who ask her to be a "surrogate" mother? When another woman receives an unsigned letter asking her to donate her eggs! When a young student boasts of being a sperm donor, every week! When a friend who tells a guy of her regret at having no children has him suggest, "Use a sperm bank!"

A colleague admitted recently that he no longer knows what to think about it all. "It's so specialized," he complained, "and so complicated." How can anyone make their way through all the technical jargon? Besides, the doctors are reassuring, infertile couples are touching, and the media serve up an array of "medical discoveries" wrapped up in fine sentiments and punctuated with photos of mothers holding their babies in their arms. So how can anyone who dares to utter a word of criticism avoid being stigmatized as an opponent of scientific progress or worse, as lacking sympathy for children or infertile couples?

How can anyone not feel uncomfortable when a friend or relative expresses a sudden yearning for a child after having postponed childbearing in order to meet the needs of career and home, because this desire, after being repressed for twenty years, resurfaces at menopause; because love, money and shared desire have never coincided; because the surgical sterilization undergone at the age of thirty now seems like a mistake; because adoption is "too complicated"; or because for a thousand other reasons they want their own baby — regardless of the risks or costs, regardless of the need to spend ten years chasing a mirage — or being led up the garden path.

When all the reasons that conception doesn't happen — infertility, sterility, a previous sterilization, the lack of a partner or one who is willing —

are presented as the same infertility problem, when technology claims to transform desires into realities, it's hard not to say: "Why not, if it's their choice?" Even though we may have a vague sense that emotions are being exploited or a sense of foreboding that what are called "personal choices" are used to mask major economic and ideological stakes, the sense of being trapped persists. Then we turn to the ethics committees, to experts and Royal commissions, hoping they will take care of the matter, set it all right, while knowing it is not really possible.

Collectively, we are slipping from the privacy of the bedroom to the chill of the laboratory, from the play of mingled bodies to the games that science plays with our bodies. We are shifting from the chance whims of love to the rigid grasp of techno-science. Our conception of human beings — both in the sense of bringing them into the world and into thought — is being shattered. We are sliding away from procreation and down a "slippery slope" leading to the industrialization of life.

And if we are left speechless by it all, it's undoubtedly because fifteen years of hammering by the media — as superficial as it is sensational — have managed to disguise fundamental concerns with minor details, and to trivialize the rest. And with such fraudulent expressions as "therapeutic" inseminations by donor or "medical indications for surrogate mothers," in use by organizations such as the Society of Obstetricians and Gynaecologists of Canada, words actually interfere with our ability to think. And it must be added that within the official debate and discussion some very basic questions have been avoided: what are the stakes, the effects, the meaning and the ultimate purpose of this new practice of manufacturing human beings?

The official discourse, as obtuse and incomplete as it is one-sided (or in many cases even false) can be summed up as follows: we are told that these techniques have been developed to "respond" to the demands of sterile couples, that they represent their last hope for having children. In the face of growing sterility, a genuine epidemic affecting (so we are told) one couple in six, how can we not be delighted at such "medical progress?" As for those who criticize the success rates, the risks, the exorbitant costs and other problems, they are brushed off as being alarmist or outmoded, while it is claimed that these "proven medical treatments" are as successful as nature. Now, admittedly, they can be a little too successful, given the number of pregnancies that produce four, five or six fetuses — or more — but some parents, so we are told, are perfectly content to have all their children at once! In other words, trust the professionals in the field, they are responsible people who have set up data banks and established the guidelines for these technologies. The final argument is that everyone has the right and the freedom to bear children. Consequently, the State should provide general access to fertility services with ethical bodies set up to provide the legitimization.

In short, if we are to believe what we are told — all is well and we can rest easy while others look after the generations yet to come — for a brave new world. But if we were to look behind the scenes...

STERILITY, MONEY, AND EXPERIMENTATION

"Should we try to improve the human species?"

"Of course."

"Genetically?"

"Of course.... We can give humankind access to a higher level of being."

These "eloquent" remarks were made by Robert Edwards who, along with Patrick Steptoe, in 1978, after ten years of unsuccessful attempts on hundreds of women, succeeded with the first *in vitro* fertilization (IVF), producing what has incorrectly been called "test-tube babies."

The interview with Edwards continues as follows:

"What are your current interests?"

"I am looking for new theories to explain how the uterus and testicles function! Why do we need the uterus?... My second research area is genetics, with a view to pre-implantation diagnosis of the human embryo. And thirdly, transplants. The cells of a nine-day-old embryo contain all the forerunners of the heart, brain, ovaries. I want to use those cells clinically: to transplant 20-day-old embryonic cells into a human brain. One day I will transplant a fetal ovary into a menopausal woman."

Edwards goes on: "We had five reasons for starting IVF: 1) to treat sterility; 2) to study trisomy (Down syndrome); 3) to carry out pre-implantation diagnosis of the human embryo; 4) to obtain embryonic cells; 5) to understand human reproduction. We've succeeded with the first points, and as far as the rest is concerned, it's just a matter of time. Today I can say quite openly what I think. In the past, I was far more cautious. We in Great Britain are coming to the end of the ethical arguments.[2] It's a battle I've been fighting for thirty years now, and I've won."[3]

Hiding behind the alibi of treating sterility, are we really talking about the use of human material for research purposes and for the quality control of children yet to be born, the entire human species? Is this simply exaggeration and boasting by an adventurous researcher? No. Robert Edwards is not the only IVF pioneer, but there is no one better situated to understand the power of the economic stakes in this sector. He is the founder of England's Bourn Hall Clinic, now part of a commercial chain of fertility clinics, teaching and research centres owned by Ares-Serono, world leader in the manufacture of pharmaceutical products used to treat infertility, with 1991 sales world-wide of $751 million and net profits of $71 million.

IVF, initially a palliative measure for fertility problems, is now used as a technique for producing embryos which can be genetically diagnosed before they are transferred to a woman's uterus. The popularity of this use of IVF was clearly in evidence at the World Conference on *in vitro* fertilization held in Paris in 1991.

The ability to bring eggs to maturity in the lab (*in vitro* maturation of oocytes), another technological offshoot of IVF, enables production of dozens of embryos at one time, and opens the way for the production of embryos destined for research and transplants. In short, we have already moved far away from the so-called "treatment of sterility!"

FROM UNSATISFIED DESIRE TO EXPERIMENTATION

How has it come about that the irrepressible desire of some people to beget children has become both the object of experimentation for some and a means of profit for others? Why has it happened so easily, so quickly — and with so few reactions?

There are five main reasons:

1. A striking opportunity to produce, inflate and over-dramatize sterility and infertility.

2. Clever rhetoric, promoted uncritically by the media, hails innovations and promotes the growth of an IVF clientele.

3. Great financial interests, and the increasing invasion of every aspect of our lives by economic values.

4. Serious gaps in ethical, scientific and social judgment affect public health priorities, strategies for training and supervision and legislation.

5. Finally, disguised behind a scientific language that fairly reeks of eugenics, is the crazy, high-stakes gamble to master and control life and its creation.

But it is not so much these individual elements (which will be discussed in detail later) that explain both our discomfort and the collective blindness that has greeted this transformation of human life. It's more the disturbing alchemical brew they boil up together; and alchemy is a fitting word for this mingling of fantasies and goals, science and dreams. Just close your eyes for a moment.

Imagine long tunnels, like arteries, that intersect and join, the way the worlds of dream and reality sometimes do. In these simultaneous worlds live people, infertile or sterile people, physicians, biologists, businessmen, lawyers, etc. Some may be anxious or in despair, others absorbed, delighted or obsessed. Each in his or her tunnel claims to be pursuing a worthy goal: for one, it's a child, for another, it's a satisfied customer, for a third, it's the attraction of prizes, grants or profits. Whatever their individual intentions, the tunnels are swept through by the force of powerful and hidden economic interests, and by the unacknowledged drive to possess and control the life of the human species, both disguised by the pretext of knowledge.

So while each person is blinded by the light at the end of her or his own tunnel, the various passions and goals are woven into a pattern none of them can yet read: the future. A future that seems already destined to be reduced to the production of "potential humans," some of them bred for research or for patent purposes — a new category, that of "infra-humans," which would shatter the very conception of humans and humanity.

If I have mixed the metaphors of alchemy, that ancestor of modern science, and of thoroughfares teeming with parallel and tangled worlds, I have done so because the reproductive technologies standing at the frontier of techno-science and ideology represent very different orders of reality, depending on what tunnel is taken and on the place that is occupied there. In this darkness, where it is so hard for each to see things clearly because our collective eyes have been hypnotized, it cannot be surprising that some will see everything in terms of a struggle against sterility, others as a question of rights and freedom, and still others as an issue of science or of money.

THE TROJAN HORSE OF STERILITY

"Sterility" is a dreadful word. Torn by fear of not being able to conceive and by the guilt at not having tried everything, how can anyone resist technologies that claim to defy the body and transform you into delighted parents? But behind the promise lies the reality: an "epidemic" of sterility both socially constructed and overestimated being used to justify the expansion of the reproductive technologies, and inflating if not infertility, then at least the number of individuals at whom these technologies are directed.

Few people are born with dysfunctional reproductive systems. For the vast majority, sterility (the inability to conceive) and infertility (delays or difficulties in doing so) are a social creation. They result either from "contraceptive" sterilization, as is the case with 40 percent of North American couples, from "medical" sterilization (removal of the uterus, ovaries, etc.), as a consequence of sexually transmitted diseases, the use of certain contraceptives and surgical procedures, or from conditions of work, life and the environment. While all these factors could be greatly reduced — and the problems of fertility along with them — the policies for prevention and detection, as well as for treatment of fertility problems, are both inadequate and inconsistent.

STERILITY: INFLATION AND CONFUSION OF TERMS

While it is often claimed that between 10 and 15 percent of couples are "sterile," the correct figure is closer to three to five percent. The higher figures, taken from a 1982 U.S. study, indicate that conception is difficult or has been delayed, not that it is impossible. These days we have the impression that it is getting harder and harder to have children. However, the data so far are clear. There has been no increase in sterility or infertility. But there is more anxiety and impatience, leading to more medical consultations, more specialists in the field and more fertility centres.

The definition of infertility widely used in the U.S. (the absence of conception after one year of sexual relations without contraception) contributes to this perception. It takes 20 percent of couples more than two years to conceive, and some as many as eight years. Moreover, some couples postpone their first child until a time when fertility is beginning to decline. It can take two years for some women to conceive after they have stopped using the contraceptive pill, although a good number of women believe that they will become pregnant as soon as they stop taking the pill — as if there was a fertility button that could be turned on and off.

In a 1990 report, the World Health Organization (WHO) suggested that infertility should be defined as no conception after two years of unprotected intercourse. WHO asks the industrialized nations to determine the prevalence of primary and secondary infertility and sterility, by gender and by cause, and strongly urges these countries to evaluate the overall medical and social options available, as well as their relative costs, rather than encourage the proliferation of the reproductive technologies.

DRAMATIZATION

Within the context of the reproductive technologies, the definition of sterility — which is often confused with infertility and now includes delays in procreation, difficulties within relationships, voluntary sterilization, and the absence or refusal of a partner — seems as elastic as the biomedical supply of these supposed remedies.

Without underestimating the problems and pain that the inability to conceive may represent, we must clarify and make less dramatic the argument that defends these technologies as the final recourse of couples desperate to have a child. A good number already have one or more children, born of one or both partners or adopted. The face of frustrated desire is not always what it seems.

Many couples who use *in vitro* fertilization have as much chance of conceiving while they're on the waiting list as from IVF. This is due both to the low success rate and to the fact that many of them are quite simply not infertile. According to a paper published by Marsden Wagner and Patricia St. Clair, 7 to 28 percent of women will conceive "naturally" before beginning IVF or in the two years after they have stopped. And an Australian report emphasizes that nine percent of couples using IVF conceived after they stopped the procedure.

AN UNSATISFIED DESIRE TRANSFORMED INTO A DISEASE

While certain pathologies or dysfunctions underlying fertility problems can be treated and cured, not conceiving cannot be considered a disease — unless we transform any frustrated desire into disease — nor should the childless be seen as people who are sick.

It is important to note that the reproductive technologies get around problems of fertility, they disguise them — but they do not cure them. A couple who are sterile before IVF will remain sterile afterwards, even if they have a child. In their case, medicine does not treat the cause, but contributes to the "manufacturing" of a child. And such a shift from "repairing" to "manufacturing" changes both the role, the definition and the status of medicine. By becoming producer, manager and user of embryos and gametes (sperm and eggs), medicine takes on unequalled power over both the individual and the social body.

Language has played an essential role in this enterprise. In fact, it is the confusion between sterility and infertility that has increased both the anxiety and the numbers of users of technology. Associating infertility and pathology has transformed technology into "therapy," to the point where even artificial insemination is sometimes described as "therapeutic." It is a verbal trick that has transformed them into "medical services" — as if procreation could be reduced to a "service" or a medical procedure! And with naming them as "medical services" comes the claim that everyone is entitled to them, with no discrimination as to marital status or sexual orientation, as if the absence or refusal of a partner were a medical problem! Verbal inflation has even led to "medical indications for the use of a surrogate mother" (see also Eichler and Sherwin in this volume), as if such a practice could be medically indicated!

Presenting these techniques in medical terms has played a major role in legitimizing them, and a good many experts in ethics and technology evaluation seem to have accepted the medical framing outright — without questioning its origins or its foundations, without questioning presuppositions or outcomes — in short being content to simply keep up after the fact as well as can be expected with sets of loose guidelines.

SERIOUS GAPS IN EVALUATION

The wait-and-see attitude on the part of those in charge is all the more surprising in view of the fact that these controversial reproductive technologies were spread in an uncontrolled manner before a full and rigorous assessment of their effectiveness, reliability, and short- and long-term safety (as well as their costs) had been carried out, a requirement still unmet 25 years after the beginnings of IVF. These technologies have become so widespread that in France, where IVF is reimbursed by the State, the number of IVF cycles started exceeds that in the United States, for a population one-quarter the size. Comparative studies of other medical options, such as tubal surgery for example, are impossible since IVF tends to be the first choice.

According to the Australian retrospective studies of Paul Lancaster, IVF is responsible for approximately 25 times the usual number of multiple births, with prenatal and neonatal mortality rates four and two times higher respectively, the risk of premature birth tripled and risks of congenital malformation doubled. The rate of very low birth-weight is 11 times higher than in the general population, with a number of babies severely handicapped as a result.

According to numerous literature reviews on the subject, especially those of Renate Klein, Patricia St. Clair and Françoise Laborie, the risks IVF poses to women are not negligible either: two to three times more spontaneous abortions, two to five times more ectopic pregnancies, 15 percent of multiple pregnancies which are triplets, quadruplets or even quintuplets, often leading to selective fetal reduction (elimination in utero of one or more fetuses). As well, these pregnancies are highly medicalized and half of them end in a cesarean. In addition, the use of ovulation-inducing drugs (so-called fertility drugs) sometimes causes nausea and ovarian cysts and, in one to two percent of cases, ovarian hyperstimulation syndrome (responsible for at least a dozen known deaths). As well, the use of the drugs is associated with an increased risk of cancers and congenital malformations.

These drugs cause the ovaries to produce many ripe follicles at one time. The eggs are "harvested" by the doctor and used to create lots of embryos which are then transferred into the uterus. Multiple embryos are necessary because it is this step, the implantation of embryos, which still accounts for 70 to 80 percent of the failures in IVF. Thus for the first time in human history, medicine has taken on the authority to produce potential human beings, described as "surplus," to offset the inefficiency of an experimental technique that has a failure rate of more than 90 percent!

The World Health Organization (WHO) emphasizes that research on these technologies has mainly been concerned with perfecting clinical protocols and broadening admissibility criteria. The WHO document states as well that this research serves the interests of those who benefit from the spread of these services, rather than assisting in rational health planning based on the real needs of the population.

FROM ECONOMIC STAKES TO FANTASY

Presented as tremendous medical feats, most of the reproductive technologies originated from techniques aimed at increasing productivity in the agricultural industry (freezing sperm and embryos, artificial insemination, ovarian stimulation, uterine lavage to transfer embryos into "carrier-cows"). Indeed, the same researchers have, in their own words, "worked weekdays on women and weekends on cows," successfully performing IVF in cattle five years after they had succeeded with women. (See Basen and Burfoot in Volume One.)

It is not so much basic research as the search for profits that lies behind these technologies. Driven by the same industrial goals of programming, performance, selection, profitability and effectiveness, they are ushering in an era of conception-on-demand with reproduction parcelled out, parents pre-selected, pregnancies fragmented, and the body being submitted to the economic and technical requirements of specialized centres. This is the implacable logic that reduces the maternal body, in contracts for child-bearing or gestation, wrongly called "surrogate mothers," to an "incubating body" — as if the status of these women had changed from that of person to that of thing. It is the same logic whereby insemination by "donor-vendor" reduces the male parent to anonymous biological material, with the doctor substituting an "inseminating pistol" for a sexual relation. Companies such as Biogenetics in the United States offer a palette of hundreds of sires, identified according to race, ethnic group, religion, colour of eyes and skin, colour and texture of hair, weight, height, bone structure, education, and occupation. The choice is tremendous — goods delivered within 24 hours, returnable within seven days! And as a bonus, quality is assured and guaranteed against AIDS.

In the same vein, some American hospitals suggest to women who are being surgically sterilized that they first undergo ovarian stimulation and then egg collection in exchange for $600 to $1000 to help defray the costs of their surgery, as well as "offering" fertility centres "new sources of eggs." Some countries are preparing to allow for the removal of the ovaries from female cadavers, to be used for the maturation of dozens of eggs and the production of as many embryos. A research program is in place in the United Kingdom to use ovaries taken from fetuses which, while never born, would still have descendants.

In the United States, Americans spend more than $2 billion on infertility treatments, with more than 80 percent of it going for pharmaceutical products. In 1987, the Office of Technology Assessment (OTA) estimated the cost of 14,000 IVF attempts at $66 million, while the artificial insemination market was evaluated at $164 million.

In Canada, most couples pay from $1500 to $4000 or more per attempt at IVF. Meanwhile, the indirect costs associated with the high rates of ectopic pregnancies, spontaneous abortions, embryonic reductions, cesareans and intensive care for newborns are assumed by the public health care system. Some people justify these exorbitant costs by comparing them with the cost of heart transplants! It is strange to compare, as some do, the symbolic death of a child that will never be, with the imminent death of an individual.

Marsden Wagner of the WHO has shown that the costs associated with the birth of a child following IVF — around $60,000 U.S. — would pay for education and information campaigns that would prevent some thirty cases of infertility! The Canadian Family Planning Federation has recently reported that since 1978 fewer women around the world have given birth to a child following IVF than become infertile every month in the United States!

I would need more space to show how these experimental, inefficient, costly practices carried out on an ethical slippery slope have achieved such importance, to the detriment of coherent prevention policies and real therapeutic interventions. More space to show how the media have contributed to shaping the collective unconscious and have too often forgone intelligent questions in favor of a sports-event model of reporting, complete with "adversaries" pitted against one another and a journalist-referee who hands out points. More space to show how the runaway events in this field have, for the most part, been supported by the experts who were supposed to analyze their validity and their effects on individuals and society. To show that the Law, which in North America is too often reduced to a utilitarian function, could have limited the temptation of omnipotence on the part of science and medicine. More space to show that by opening the Pandora's box of embryo and gamete manipulation, these procreation technologies are becoming part of the bio-revolution of the 21st century along with mega-projects for mapping the human genome.

To conclude, some observations by psychoanalyst Monette Vacquin.

It is a stunning paradox that today, the generation which came after Nazism is giving the world tools for eugenics that go far beyond Hitler's wildest dreams.... The scientists of tomorrow will have a power that exceeds all the powers hitherto known to humankind: the power to manipulate the human genome. Who can swear that it will only be used to avoid hereditary diseases? Some are coldly asking for the rational mastery and perfection of the human genetic heritage. Others, haunted by a sense of menace, remembering the radically different origins of wisdom and science, think that perhaps legitimate intentions to cure carry within them other deeply hidden forces, which are beyond control. Relief of suffering, the physician's task, seems to have been transformed into an exorbitant duty to cure all humankind. But of what? The human condition too is a hereditary disease — and it is sexually transmitted!"

NOTES

This text was initially published in the September 1992 issue of the *Revue Notre Dame*, a free monthly magazine with a very large distribution in Quebec. It is the policy of this publication not to include footnotes or bibliographies with the articles (although some notes have been added for this book). This piece is based largely on my previous work, especially my Ph.D. thesis and research projects funded by the Social Sciences and Humanities Research Council (SSHRC).

1 *La Presse*, August 12, 1992.

2 In 1990, The British Government passed the Human Embryology Act giving scientists a green light to carry out reproductive and genetic experimentation.

3 Gauthier, U., "Voyage chez les sorciers de la vie. Va-t-on modifier l'espèce humaine?," *Le Nouvel Observateur*, Doc. no. 10, 1990.

BIBLIOGRAPHY

Ambroselli, Claire, "Quarante ans après le Code de Nuremberg: éthique médicale et droits de l'homme," *Éthique médicale et droits de l'homme*, Actes Sud/INSERM, avril 1988, pp. 19-40.

Bolton, Virginia, Osborn, John, Servante, Denise, "The human fertilisation and embryology act 1990 — A British case history for legislation on bioethical issues," *Journal International. Bioéthique*, vol. 3, no. 2, 1992, pp. 95-101.

Burstyn, Varda, "Making babies," "Making perfect babies" in *Canadian Forum*, Ottawa, March/April 1992.

Corea, Gena, *The Mother Machine*, New York, Harper & Row, 1985, p. 374.

De Vilaine, Anne-Marie, Gavarinl, L., et M. Le Coadic, (eds), *Maternité en mouvement. Les femmes la reproduction et les hommes de science*, Grenoble, Presse de l'Université de Grenoble et Montréal, Ed. Saint-Martin,1986, p. 244.

Decorney Jacques, "De l'irresponsabilité mortelle à la vraie maîtrise de la vie," *Le monde diplomatique. L'Homme en danger de science?*, Manière de voir 15, May 1992, p. 24-27; "Un temps pour réfléchir," *Le monde diplomatique*, Manière de voir 15, mai 1992, p. 96-97.

Duelli-Klein, Renate, et Robyn Rowland "Women as test-sites for fertility drugs: Clomiphene citrate and hormonal cocktails," *Reproductive and Genetic Engineering, Journal of International Feminist Analysis*, Pergamon Press, Vol. 1, No 3, 1988, pp. 251-275.

Dufresne, Jacques, *La reproduction humaine industrialisée*, Québec, Institut Québécois de recherche sur la culture,1986, p. 125.

Gavarini, Laurence "Les 'biomédiateurs': une nouvelle figure entre le médico-social et l'eugénisme" pp.213-225 *Actes du Colloque L'enceinte des technologies de procréation*, 57e Congrès de l'ACFAS, L.

Hermitte, M.-A., "F.I.V. et tri des embryons," *Génétique et Liberté*, Jan.-Feb. 1992, pp. 4-5.

Klein, Renate, [ed.] *Infertility, Women speak out about their experience on reproductive medicine*, Pandora Press, 1989, p. 328.

Laborie, Françoise, "Nouvelles technologies de la reproduction (NTR): risques pour la santé des enfants," *Actes du colloque de l'Association internationale des démographes de langue française*, Delphes, 6-10 October 1992, p. 7.

Lauzon Léo-Paul, "Un remède anti-dépression financière," *Le Devoir*, 26-27 June 1993, p. A-9.

Limoges, Camille, "L'Évaluation sociale des technologies et ses tâches," *Actes du Colloque Les pratiques de l'évaluation sociale des technologies*, Conseil de la science et de la technologie, Québec, 1991;

"Éthique médicale et évaluation sociale des technologies," *Éthique médicale et droits de l'homme*, Actes Sud/INSERM, April 1988 b, pp. 307-312.

Marcus-Steiff, Joachim, "La mesure des taux de "succès" de la FIV (fécondation *in vitro* et transfert d'embryon)," *Actes du Colloque de l'Association internationale des démographes de langue française*, Delphes, 6-10 October 1992, p. 13.

Nali, Jean-Yves, "Grossesses sur ordonnance," *Le Monde*, June 23, 1993, p. 19.

OMS, Regional Office for Europe, *Consultation on the Place of in vitro Fertilization in Infertility Care*, Copenhagen, 18-22 June 1990, Summary Report, p. 7.

Raymond, Janice G., "At issue: of eggs, embryos and altruism," *Reproductive and Genetic Engineering*, Journal of International Feminist Analysis, Pergamon Press, Vol. 1, No 3, 1988, pp. 281-286.

RCNTR "Royal Commission on New Reproductive Technologies," *Press Kit, Fertility Programs in Canada*, April 1993, Ottawa.

Rowland, Robyn, *Living Laboratories: Women and Reproductive Technologies*, Bloomington and Indianapolis, Indiana University Press, 1992, p. 366.

Rutnam, Romaine, "Evaluating *in vitro* fertilization technology in Australia," *Community Health Studies*, vol. XIV, no. 3, 1990.

SOGC, "Considérations déontologiques sur les nouvelles techniques de reproduction. VIII: Banques de sperme et utilisation des gamètes et des embryons," Rapport du comité de la SOGC, *Journal SOGC*, April 1993, p. 324.; "Ethical considerations of the new reproductive technologies," rapport du comité de la SOGC, *Journal SOGC*, June 1993, p. 643; "Reproductive Toxicology," clinical interview, *Journal SOGC*, April 1993, p. 306.

St. Clair Stephenson, "The risks associated with ovulation induction," *Iatrogenics*, vol. 1, 1991, pp.7-16.

Stephens, Thomas and McLean Janice, with Rona Achilles, Lucie Brunet and Janis Wood Catano, *Enquêtes sur les programmes d'infertilité au Canada*, Commission royale sur les nouvelles techniques de reproduction, April 1993.

Testart Jacques, "La perversion de l'idéal de recherche", *Le monde diplomatique. L'Homme en danger de science?*, Manière de voir 15, mai 1992a, p. 18-20; (ed.) *Le magasin des enfants*, Paris, Editions François Bourin, 1990, 338 p; "À la recherche du cobaye idéal," *Le monde diplomatique. L'Homme en danger de science?*, Manière de voir May 15, 1992b, p. 82-85; *Le désir du gène*, Paris, Editions François Bourin, 1992c, p. 281.

Tort, Michel, "Le traitement psychologique de la demande d'enfant dans la procréation artificielle," *Psychanalyse à l'Université*, Vol. 12, No. 46, April 1987.

Tougas, Claudette, "Les retard inexcusables de la Commission Baird," éditorial, *La Presse*, July 8 1993.

Trépannier Isabelle, *La fécondation in vitro et transfert d'embryons: traitement ou expérimentation? Le cas de cinq rapports nationaux*: Warnock, Brenda, 5 Sages, MSSS, et Lenoir, *Mémoire de maîtrise en sociologie*, UQAM, May, 1993.

Vacquin Monette, *Frankenstein ou les délires de la raison*, Éd. François Bourin, 1989, p. 230.

Vandelac, L., "Commission Baird: rigueur du processus de recherche ou secret de rigueur?" *Interface*, Vol 14, no 2 March-April 1993; "Dispositifs d'évaluation des technologies de reproduction: évaluation éthique, Technology Assessment et évaluation sociale: éléments d'analyse critique." *Actes du Colloque, Deuxième Symposium international de Martigny sur la fertilité, Changements dans le processus de la reproduction humaine: aspects médicaux et démographiques*. March 20-21, 1992 b), Martigny, Suisse. *A paraître dans Congrès et Colloques de l'INED*, Presses universitaires de France; "Embryons congelés: derrière la glace d'une certaine éthique biomédicale" pp. 259-287, in *Contribution à la réflexion bioéthique*, Dialogue France-Québec, Durand, Guy et Cartherine Perrotin (éds.) *Actes du Colloque Ethique biomédicale*, "Troisièmes Entretiens" du Centre Jacques Cartier, Lyon 1991, Ed., Fides, Mlt. 1991, p. 315; "Fertile stérilité ou l'infertilité idiopathique entre le réel et l'imaginaire..." *Sexualité et Infertilité, Actes du Colloque Infertilité et sexualité*, 58e Congrès de l'ACFAS, WMC Brown, Iowa, 1992 c), p. 90; "Technologies de procréation: du redéploiement de la médecine a l'emprise du biopouvoir," pp. 243-260, *Du privé au politique: la maternité et le travail comme enjeux des rapports de sexes. De l'expérience de la maternité à l'enceinte des technologies de procréation*. Vandelac, L., et Al. (Textes réunis par) Publications GIERF/CRF, UQAM, October 1990 a, p. 428; "Technologies de reproduction: techniques de régulation à la hausse ou véritables montagnes russes?" *Actes du Colloque de l'Association internationale des démographes de langue française*, Delphes, Oct. 6-10 1992a A paraître; Vandelac, L., et Al. (Textes réunis par), *Du privé au politique: la maternité et le travail comme enjeux des rapports de sexes. De l'expérience de la maternité à l'enceinte des technologies de procréation. Actes de la Section d'études féministes du 57e Congrès de l'ACFAS*, Publications GIERF/CRF, UQAM, October 1990c p. 428; *L'infertilité et la stérilité: l'alibi des technologies de procréation, Thèse de sociologie, Doctorat nouveau régime (Ph.D.)*, Université Paris VII, Jussieu, May 1988 a, p. 504; "La face cachée de la procréation artificielle," *La Recherche*, No 213, pp. 1112-1124, Spécial La sexualité, Sept. 1989, Paris.; "Technologies de procréation et 'biologisation' de la paternité," pp. 241-250, *Actes de la table ronde internationale de l'APRE (Atelier production-reproduction), Rapports sociaux de sexes: Problématiques, méthodologies, champs d'analyse*, CNRS, Paris 24-26 nov. 87, mai 1988b, p. 274; "Vulgarisation entre scientisme et sensationalisme: la presse "enceinte" des mères porteuses," pp. 246-275 dans D. Jacobi et B. Schiele (eds), *Vulgariser la science, ou le procès de l'ignorance*, Paris, Editions Champ Vallon, (coll. Milieux) mai 1988 c), p. 284.

Vandelac, L., McTeer, M., Hébert, M. et B. Hatfield, "Passer le "bébé" au prochain gouvernement? Fignoler l'emballage du rapport de $26 millions? Ou profiter des vacances de juillet pour noyer le poisson et éviter les vagues?" Les ex-commissaires condamnent la deuxième prolongation de mandat de la Commission Royale sur les nouvelles technologies de reproduction. *Le Droit*, Ottawa, Nov. 17, 1992, *La Presse*, Montréal, Nov. 18, 1992

PART V

WOMEN AS GESTATORS; CHILDREN AS PRODUCTS

Among the many themes implicit in the proliferation of all the new reproductive and genetic technologies (NRGTs) is the commercialization of pregnancy, a view of women and children as objects, of women as "gestators," children as "products." Reading the papers in this section brings this theme to light, exposing the dangers of this approach for women, for children, for all of us.

Multiple births and prematurity are frequent when the new reproductive technologies are applied. We may smile at the triplets we pass in their strollers, marvel at the wonders of modern medicine that maintain the most fragile young lives, but what is it like to be the parents of these children? Personal testimony, too long marginalized as only of anecdotal interest by most male academics, needs to be included in any discussion of the impact of biomedical technologies, and the chapters by Donna

Launslager, Laura Sky and Lisa Mitchell make the problems, the pain and the paradoxes in their use a vivid reality.

Clearly, however, the legal system is not prepared for these realities, this subjectivity of pregnancy, childbirth and childrearing. The legal system certainly does not give these realities legitimacy when it ignores what it means to give "informed consent" (Karen Capen) when outcomes are unknown and so much that is experimental is touted as treatment. It ignores the experience of pregnancy when courts increasingly view women as at odds with the children they are carrying (Ronda Bessner), as if a woman with a pregnancy she wants can be separated from it.

And, through increasing social practices, too, with the commissioning of women and the contracting of pregnancies (Margrit Eichler, Susan Sherwin) as well as with biomedically creating postmenopausal pregnancies (Abby Lippman), women become containers, vessels, objects for gestating, mere systems in which children can be produced.

From the personal to the political, the new reproductive and genetic technologies — all biomedical technologies — are reshaping parenthood. And these shapes are not just concepts, but living, vital women and children as portrayed in the pages that follow.

24

Donna Launslager

As the mother of quadruplets, I have learned firsthand what it means for a parent suddenly to have several newborns added to the family. The physical, psychological and financial pressures are unimaginable. Our transformation from a small unit of two parents with a toddler to a family of seven was completely unexpected. I had not taken fertility drugs and there was no family history of multiple births.

My husband, David, and I felt overwhelmed by the prospect of caring for four additional babies in our modest house, especially when we realized that there was no support system for parents in our situation through government programs or social services. At first, we couldn't even find a grass-roots organization that could help with advice and access to private and volunteer resources.

REMEMBERING

I remember clearly the day that the ultrasound technician in the hospital told us that we were expecting quadruplets. David and I were overwhelmed with questions. How could this possibly happen to us? There was no history of multiple births on either side of the family. I was not receiving infertility treatment. Thirty-one years old at the time, I had a history of spontaneous abortions prior to the birth of our son, who was then 15 months old. With this background, how was I going to carry these babies long enough for all to be healthy? How could I deal emotionally with losing one or more of these babies? If they all survived, how was

I going to be able to spread my love over four babies plus a two-year-old? Since these babies were at high risk of being born prematurely and of having low birth-weight, what if one or more were born with disabilities? What if one or more of them needed to stay in the hospital for a long time? Would we then be able to visit them and also care for the others at home? How was little Michael going to cope with us bringing home four newborns?

Naturally, one of us would have to give up our job to take care of these children, but how could we meet all these new commitments on one income? How could we safely fit five infant car seats into our five-passenger vehicle — and remain within the law? If we couldn't, could we afford to buy a new van? Our small three-bedroom bungalow was not large enough for seven, but could we afford to build an addition? Without relatives nearby to give us a hand, how were we going to cope? How could we afford the help we would need? If David could get a teaching job closer to home, would he give up his seniority and start at a new school board on a temporary contract?

Looking for answers to all these important questions made for a very stressful pregnancy. We had no one to turn to for guidance, since we were the only family in the Hamilton-Wentworth area that had gone through this experience. My obstetrician and other care givers offered us very little support other than a prescription for iron and calcium. They did offer us the services of a social worker, but we didn't need someone to sit and talk to. What we needed was "hands on" and financial help, and that was unavailable. Yet somehow I had faith that everything would work out all right.

Even though our families lived far away, it gave us strength to know that they were there for us with emotional support. It was also comforting to know that the people from our small community were ready to help. Early in my pregnancy I received a call from a retired maternity nurse who offered to organize a team of volunteers to help us with the babies when they came home from the hospital. We were very grateful for this offer, but the thought of having a troop of strangers passing through our home each day was almost as overwhelming as the thought of having four babies at once. So we decided that we would try to manage the work-load ourselves.

Our babies were born at 36 weeks — all four of them healthy and weighing from two-and-a-half to just under five pounds. Two were identical and two fraternal. Being the first set of quadruplets at McMaster University Medical Centre, they had made medical history. This resulted in a certain notoriety and media attention, which we found very uncomfortable. After going through such an emotionally and physically exhausting birth, we found the media aggressiveness very stressful. However, we finally agreed to participate in a press conference, with hopes that this would lead to corporate donations of formula, food, diapers, clothing and equipment from infant product companies.

A few companies came forward with donations. One donated a supply of infant formula. Another provided a six-month supply of disposable diapers and a few small companies and community groups donated clothing and equipment. These donations, though, were not given because of media attention but because caring individuals contacted companies on our behalf. The only attention we received as a result of the media was a few crank calls from strangers. One caller pretended to be a nurse in the hospital, calling to say that all four babies had died. This frightening experience made us extremely cautious and forced us to re-evaluate any future media contacts.

Two weeks after my release from the hospital, two of the babies came home. Since David needed to be alert for his work, it was impossible for him to help with night feedings. After just one week of handling the feedings of two babies along with caring for Michael plus continuing visits to see the other two babies in the hospital, I quickly became physically exhausted. At this time, I realized that we did in fact need the help of volunteers.

It seemed like the entire town of Caledonia responded to our needs. Thirty-two volunteers came to our rescue and helped with the daily routines, feedings, bathing and outings in two tandem strollers. Many were senior citizens who, to our surprise, were grateful for being needed. People said that the birth of our babies brought out a generous spirit in our community. Without their help we could not have maintained a sane household.

We were very concerned about Michael. To make sure that he wouldn't feel shunned, I took him to a neighbor's home where he played with their children while the volunteers and I were taking care of the quadruplets. I think we almost overcompensated so that he wouldn't be neglected. Fortunately, he is extremely well adjusted and from the beginning felt protective of his brother and sisters.

People automatically assumed that I had taken fertility drugs, and nine times out of ten they freely asked about it. I got the impression that the general opinion is, "Okay, you took these drugs and knew the risks, so don't come looking for help now." But you get inured to these kinds of remarks. When I told people that I had never taken fertility drugs, they would look wide-eyed and say, "Oh my god, I'm glad it's you and not me." And I always replied, "I'm glad it's me, too."

Our small house was bursting at the seams. We had all four babies in one bedroom and our single-car garage had been transformed into a warehouse for formula, diapers, donated clothing, strollers and equipment. But we needed more space. After much consideration, we decided that David would seek other employment and we would buy a larger house in our home town to be closer to our families. When our babies were five months old, we moved and said good-bye to our 32 wonderful volunteers who had become very good friends.

The child-related expenses we incurred during the first few months were $11,000 above what it would have cost us to have a single baby. Aside from that, we lost my income, traded in our small car for a seven-passenger vehicle and bought a larger home. Financial planning and budgeting was and continues to be of the utmost importance. We purchased second-hand clothing and equipment, borrowed layette equipment whenever possible, and diapers, baby food and other needs were bought in bulk or on special sales whenever possible. When the babies had outgrown their clothing and equipment, we sold these items to offset new expenses.

When our four little ones turned two years old, it was becoming apparent that the single most limiting factor in bringing up multiple birth children is time. There is simply less time for teaching, training, playing and taking care of the individual needs of each child. Even with two to three hours of help in the home every day, time is still in short supply.

Organization and strict scheduling have been the key to our survival. All of our babies were fed and bathed at the same time. Diapers were changed at set times, and the babies followed the same sleeping schedule whether they liked it or not. When they were infants, charts were kept to ensure that we didn't forget to feed one of them and we also noted down bowel movements. At age two, they were all toilet trained at the same time. Clothing, toys and soothers were colour coded to avoid confusion.

Since the birth of our three daughters and son, in March 1985, I have learned the outer limits of one's capacity to parent and we have learned to gratefully accept help from many sources. Eventually, after we settled into a stable, though hectic, family routine, it seemed natural that I offer my support to others who were going through the same experience. Because of my concern about the lack of awareness among health providers, government and the general public around multiple births issues — preconceptional, prenatal, postnatal and childhood years — I became deeply involved as a volunteer with the Parents of Multiple Births Association of Canada (P.O.M.B.A.). In my new-found role as a lobbyist for this growing self-help group which now has 60 affiliates, I am involved in offering peer support to over 5,000 families with twins, triplets and higher order multiples across Canada.

MULTIPLE BIRTHS: FACTS AND FIGURES

Statistics Canada figures indicate that since 1974, twin births have risen 35 percent, triplet births have doubled and quadruplet births increased by 400 percent.[1] Due to inadequate statistics and poor reporting methods in the past, the data do not give the exact number of triplets, quadruplets or quintuplets that have been born alive, how many were stillborn or how many survived within a set. Neither do we know the number of fetuses lost prior to 20 weeks gestation.

Prior to 1987, the only quintuplet birth registered in Canada was of the famous Dionne Quints, who were removed from their parents at birth and cared for by social services because the parents were deemed incapable of caring for the five infants. Since 1987, six sets of quintuplets have been born in Canada, all through the use of reproductive technologies. I have learned the facts behind the epidemic of triplet and higher order multiple births in western countries brought about by the widespread use of fertility treatments through my work with P.O.M.B.A. Data show that women over 34 years of age are at higher risk of spontaneously conceiving multiples, just as they are more likely to receive fertility assistance, which also puts them at a higher risk of multiple births.

A multiple birth may seem attractive after years of infertility, but people receiving fertility treatment should be made aware of the implications of giving birth to two, three, four or five babies at once. Yet Canadian fertility clinics give little or no counselling on the emotional and financial ramifications of a multiple birth. Information is limited to the fertility procedure itself. People seeking new reproductive technologies should be completely informed about the implications of their treatment so that they can take full responsibility for their lives.

Worldwide research on multiple births reveal the following facts:

*Approximately 10 percent of all perinatal deaths are multiple birth babies.[2]

*Disabilities are over five times more common in multiple-birth children than single children.[3]

*Children in multiple-birth families are 2 1/2 times more likely to be victims of child abuse.[4]

*Parents of multiples are under multiple mental, physical and financial stresses from expecting and caring for the babies. They are at higher than average risk for drug and alcohol abuse, family violence and divorce.[5]

*Multiple birth babies are at higher risk for both immediate and long-term health problems.

*Multiple birth babies are more likely to be admitted to neonatal intensive care units after birth. With increasing numbers, the birth weight of each baby decreases and the need for special and intensive care increases.

*Multiple-births provide a disproportionately high number of children with special needs requiring expensive extra educational support.

*A high percentage of triplets and higher order multiple births are conceived through infertility treatments which in some provinces are paid for by provincial health insurance plans.[6]

*A multiple pregnancy carries far more risk for a woman than a single one.

*Women expecting multiples are often admitted into hospitals for long periods, increasing stress on the family and costs to the health care system.

*Prenatal nutrition is important to improve a multiple-birth outcome yet specialized nutritional education is given to few women expecting multiples[7],

*Families with multiple-birth children, especially families with triplets and higher order multiple-births, face extraordinary expenses which can cause financial disaster. Families with an average income who have multiples born to them can find themselves reduced to financial poverty.

WORKING FOR CHANGE

As Health and Education Director of P.O.M.B.A., I have been lobbying for changes in government policies to assist families with multiples. A 1983 Australian study clearly illustrated the impossibility of coping without help from outside the family.[8] The data revealed that for the first six months of the infants' lives, parents provide an average of 197.5 hours of care per week (recall that there are but 168 hours in a week). This is usually provided by the mother, the main caregiver, who has her own needs in these hours to bathe, dress, sleep, eat, relax or just talk to her husband. It is obvious that the parents who are unable to employ homemaking services must rely on family or volunteer help to maintain a sane household.

At P.O.M.B.A., our first lobbying effort was aimed at provincial governments across Canada. We requested an extension of homemaking programs to include families with triplets, quadruplets and quintuplets. Our plan was to start with the Ontario Ministry of Community and Social Services, Ontario being the province with the most multiple births. Our request was denied. The Minister in charge, Charles Beer, replied that "the Integrated Homemaker program is intended to assist only the frail elderly and adult physically disabled people and therefore we are not prepared to extend the program to serve multiple birth families." The Minister suggested that families with multiples seek help through their local Home Support Program at a user fee of $7 per hour.

It became evident that if both the mother and the birth babies were well upon release from the hospital, families with multiples fell between the cracks of all government subsidized homemaker programs. With universal programs being phased out, governments are not prepared to expand any family services.

Our next strategy was to approach the Federal Government. We requested that parents of triplets and higher order multiples pay reduced income tax to accommodate child care expenses and other extraordinary costs. Our research showed that a high percentage of families with triplet and higher order multiple births did not qualify for child care expense deductions because they were single-income families. The Federal Government's deduction on personal income tax is $4,000.00 per child, given exclusively to double-income families who use formal day care facilities that offer tax receipts. Clearly, this benefit is not tied to need. The Federal Government has also introduced a claw-back feature on Family Allowance Benefits to families with a single income exceeding $50,000.00, while leaving untouched the family allowance benefits of families with two incomes of $49,999.00 each.

We soon realized the importance of rallying the support of other organizations who shared our concerns about tax, health and social issues. We first collaborated with the Canadian Institute of Child Health in a proposal to the Royal Commission on New Reproductive Technologies, asking that they initiate studies to collect information on a number of medical, social, economic and ethical concerns related to higher order multiple births. Our request was declined. The Royal Commission did indicate, however, that they intended to recommend measures to reduce the likelihood of multiple births arising from fertility drugs and fertility clinics.

LESSONS LEARNED

Through international links with other multiple birth organizations, such as the International Society of Twin Studies in Rome, Italy, we have gained new understanding of multiple birth issues and the services that are offered abroad. Governments and researchers in other countries are dealing with the same issues that concern us here, including the controversial issues about the moral and ethical dilemmas that are associated with reproductive technologies. In Canada there are, for example, no guidelines or safeguards in place to regulate the use of fertility drugs like Pergonal and Clomiphene. Similarly, Canada has not dealt with issues such as the number of multiple fertilized eggs to implant to insure successful *in vitro* fertilization without the risks of a pregnancy involving three, four, five or six fetuses. Nor has Canada faced the implications of the medical procedure of "selective reduction" in a multiple pregnancy and, if this were to be allowed, what number of fetuses should be reduced, when and how.

Meanwhile the numbers of multiples are growing. According to Statistics Canada, there are currently over 100,000 multiple-birth children in Canada under the age of 13, with 41,000 of these five years and under. Each year the country adds 8,300 twin babies and 270 babies in triplets, quadruplets and quintuplets. Although these multiple babies represent only 2 percent of all births, they account for 16 percent of the low birth-weight infant population. Statistics Canada also reports that almost half of all twins and over 93 percent of triplets and higher order multiple births are born prematurely and of low birth-weight.[9]

It is a continuing challenge to get governments' attention concerning the many problems associated with multiple births, especially with current financial restraints. Whenever possible, Federal and Provincial health programs are being moved from a hospital setting to community-based health and care programs. They are looking to grass-roots organizations like P.O.M.B.A. to fill the gaps in services they cannot provide.

Low birth-weight and prematurity have fortunately remained priority health issues and are on the agenda of Canadian governments at all levels. This has given us the opportunity to promote the awareness of multiple-birth issues by linking up with the Low Birth Weight and Prematurity Prevention Coalition, an alliance of government, voluntary organizations and health professionals under the umbrella of the Canadian Institute of Child Health.

Looking back on my life as a mother of five and an advocate for Canadian multiple birth families, I feel privileged that I can add my voice to those of other multiple birth parents.

REFERENCES

1   Millar W.J., Wadhera S, Nimrod C: *Multiple Births: Trends and Patterns in Canada 1974-1990*. *Health Reports* (Statistics Canada, Cat. 82-003), 1992; 4(3):223-250.

2   Botting B, MacDonald-Davis I, MacFarlane A: "Recent trends in the incidence of multiple-births and their mortality." *Arch Dis Child;* 62-941-50, 1987.

3   Simpson H, Walker G: "Estimate of the costs required for neonatal intensive care." *Arch Dis Child;* 56-90, 1981.

4   Nelson H, Martin C: *Increased Child Abuse In Twins*. A Report from the Department of Psychiatry, Lexington, Kentucky: University of Kentucky Medical Centre, 1985.

5   Parents of Multiple Births Association of Canada's survey: *Impact of Multiples on the Family*, 1991.

6   Botting B, MacFarlane A, Price F: *Three, Four and More. A Study of Triplets and Higher Order Births*. London: HMSO, 1990.
     Baird P: *Reproductive Technology and Child Health*. Presented at Child Health 2000. A World Congress and Exposition on Child Health, Vancouver, February 22, 1992, Royal Commission on New Reproductive Technologies, Ottawa, 1992.
7   Dubois S, Dougherty C, Duquette MP: "Twin pregnancy: The impact of the Higgins nutrition intervention program on maternal and neonatal outcomes," *Am J Clin Nutr* 1991;53:1397-1403.
8   Stewart P, Hennessy J: *A report on the investigation of the social and economic disadvantage of triplet families*. University of NSW Sydney, Department of Sociology, Sydney, Australia, 1983.
9   Millar W.J., Wadhera S, Nimrod C: *Multiple Births: Trends and Patterns in Canada 1974-1990*. *Health Reports* (Statistics Canada, Cat. 82-003), 1992; 4(3):223-250.

25

TO HURT AND TO HEAL

Laura Sky

In her film, To Hurt and To Heal, film maker Laura Sky brings us face to face with the complex issues raised by another set of medical technologies — those found in the neonatal intensive care units of modern hospitals.

Part one of the film is an uncut interview with Gaylene and Bill Levesque. Although their baby was not born after infertility treatment, their experiences are like those of many others whose babies were born after IVF and other reproductive interventions. We present an abridged version of that interview.

INTERVIEW

GAYLENE: My water broke when I was in my 25th week of pregnancy and so I went to the hospital and at first they told us that there was no hope, that the baby would be delivered dead. When we sort of started dealing with that, they came in and said that they'd talked to the doctors in the neonatal unit and that they felt that there might be a chance. Which really excited us a lot, it gave us a kind of hope that, well, that we hadn't really expected. And when I went into labour and the baby was delivered, I still couldn't conceive of the fact that he would be born alive. When he was delivered we heard this little tiny cry, like a little mew and then the doctors and nurses from neonatal rushed in like a bunch of robots, it looked like to me, and grabbed him and started working on him. I could see this little movement going up and down. It was his leg kicking and I remember we looked at each other and we said he's alive, he's alive. We were just so thrilled with this whole thought that there was life there.

I had talked to the doctor from neonatal before our son was born and I said I don't want any heroic measures. I would like nature to determine whether our son lives or not. And he said no, no heroic measures. Then I walked into that neonatal unit and I said my God this whole place is heroic measures! Those lights were just so bright and the noise level was so high and I felt really disturbed by that because I knew that the baby was so used to being comforted, with the sound muffled and that it was nice and dark, and I thought this must be very hard for him. We were really shocked by what we saw because there was this tiny perfect infant and there were tubes and things all over the place.

They told us that the first 72 hours would be the telling point — whether he would live or not — and so those hours were really torture for us. But I guess it was the third day he looked a lot better and I noticed when I walked into the neonatal unit that people, they smiled at me for the first time. Before, everybody would look at me very concerned and suddenly everybody smiled at me. Then the doctors said they wanted to talk to me. I thought they were going to congratulate me on this wonderful thing. This baby was going to live. Instead, they told us that he had suffered a very severe brain hemorrhage and that... that it was the most serious bleed that was possible — they called it a grade four bleed and that this meant that the child would more than likely be very severely... handicapped was the term they used. And they wanted me to call Bill in so that we could discuss it.

BILL: This type of neonatal unit was still so new that a lot of the long-term effects and things, they weren't sure of. So I can remember, at the time, not really realising the consequences for the future.

They would always have options. They would say, well he had this grade four bleed, but we have no idea what effect this will have. So you always have the positive option that it won't be a major effect on him and you go through with that. And then when something else goes wrong and you're kind of devastated again, and then you start adjusting to that, and you say okay, we can survive that, we'll live with that, he's alive. And then another setback will occur and then you're back down again. So in a short time you're experiencing so much emotional trauma that you just can't believe that it's only been a couple of days. You think that oh, it's been going on for months and the time span is so short, abbreviated.

GAYLENE: When I heard about this grade four bleed, the first thing I said to Bill was what's this going to mean to our future and to the future of our other children? I mean are we going to have a child who can't sit up, can't feed himself, can never talk, can never do anything? And what effect is this going to have on our lives? And Bill is always thinking short-term and he said yeah but he's alive and we're going to go with that. And I'm saying yeah, but what kind of life is this? Not just for him, but for... for all of us. And I found that was most difficult time because I was imagining the future, you know. I was saying what's going to happen when our daughter says can you come watch me play basketball? And I say no we can't go because how can we find a babysitter? Or a 17 year old who can't go to the bathroom by himself and that sort of stuff. I remember saying to Bill too, oh it's okay for you, you're going to go out to work every day. This is going to be like the end of my life. I'm going to have to devote my life to this and it was a really selfish kind of thing but it was, to be honest, my immediate reaction.

BILL: Well, I tended to concentrate on the short-term because I found that was a way for me to cope with it. I thought about the long-term occasionally. We had told the doctors that we didn't need any heroic measures, but neither of us defined what we meant by heroic measures. So they were probably pretty well doing heroic measures. I didn't realize they were, and I didn't realize what the ultimate consequences were. They would give you some ideas, but I wasn't very clear on exactly what was down the road. So I was just mainly concentrating on the day to day surviving.

GAYLENE: It seemed to us that when the severity of the bleed is so great my first feeling was that we should discontinue treatment, all treatment. Bill didn't like that option at all and it was something that we sat and we discussed for a long time. And finally we came to what we felt was a... a legitimate compromise, and we asked the doctors to return so we could discuss this with them. And our compromise, perhaps to a medical person may sound silly, but it was what we could cope with at the time. We said that we wanted was that there be an opportunity, the term I used was, for God to have some say in this whole thing.

To tell us, to somehow guide us as to what should happen next. So what we suggested as a compromise was that the life support systems, the respirator, be kept on, and that IV feedings be continued but that no other treatments be done. That anything that came up not be treated so that we could see whether he was going to rally, or if he was going to go into decline. That was what we agreed on. And the doctors seemed to find that option agreeable too. They said fine.

I remember you [speaking to Bill] saying at the time something to the effect that you felt if we'd taken him off we somehow would have been responsible for, for not giving him a chance, somehow that we'd have been responsible for him dying.

BILL: Yeah, I wanted to go as far as I felt I could, and see if Jean André [their son] could take it from there somewhere along the line.

GAYLENE: He was so tiny and so young and I remember putting my little finger in the palm of his hand. He would squeeze my finger and it would just make me feel like on top of the world. You know there's that connection and there was life and he could do that. And then I'd walk out and I'd think am I going to feel this happy about it when he's 18 and that's still the only reaction I can get from him? And then I try and put that out of my mind.

The thing is, we thought we made it very clear, we didn't want anything treated. We wanted nature to take its course, while still giving him the chance to fight back. And then I walked in one day and they were all surrounding him and they were resuscitating him and I said, "What's going on here? I thought we had made it clear we didn't want this kind of thing going on." And they said, "Oh well, you know it wasn't really him, it was the machine that malfunctioned, and we're not really doing what you think we're doing." And then we were in another time and we saw that they were treating, they were giving him antibiotics, and I said, "What are you giving him? Is that food?" And they said "No it's antibiotics." And I said, "What for?" And they said, "Well, you know he has a kidney infection." I said, "Well, time to talk to the doctors again." So we called the doctors and we talked to the doctors again and this time they said, "Well you know we don't consider this heroic measures, this sort of cropped up and we just deal with it. It's just an infection, it wouldn't really kill him, it would just hurt him." I started getting a little uneasy. I started thinking, "It was torment for us to make this decision in the first place. We spent literally hours talking about it and trying to get down to our souls to make this kind of decision. And then presenting it to them is the most difficult thing we've ever done. And then it felt like it had just been a game to them. They didn't care what we thought. They were just treating him.

BILL: We just didn't understand what they meant by heroic measures, and what we meant by heroic measures.

GAYLENE: The neonatal unit itself scared me. It was so unreal. I mean those incredibly bright bright lights. And it was so hot. I had just given birth and I was a little weak and I would often feel like I was going to faint there, you know. And the noise level was so high that it would irritate me. And then all these machines, and all the noises the machines made. And of course alarms were always going off, and people would be rushing here and there. And all these things sticking into my baby, and he looked so uncomfortable and at one point they had to tape down his arms and legs so that he wouldn't move, because the movement would disrupt the machinery. To me the whole thing was heroic measures.

You know they would say something to me like, "Oh well, this happens with babies like this all the time, and we can do this but we can't do that." And I would think, "They know they can't do that because they've done it to other babies and other babies have died." That's how they know. They say, "We have to be very careful with the dosage because we can only give this much 'cause that much will do this, and that much will do that. And I think, "How many babies had to die before they found that out?" I sort of felt like it was a sacrifice going on here; that I should be thankful that all these babies went through it; and at the same time I was almost mourning those other babies that had to lose their lives just so they could get Jean André to this point.

BILL: You're thinking of what the ultimate effects will be for the baby, and yet you don't want to make the decision to end it all. I mean you have to live with that the rest of your life. Could he have made it? Did I do the wrong thing? So you wait for the doctor to kind of get the ball rolling, that we're getting pretty well to the point where we can't do too much more. So that you could say, "Well then, let's stop the heroic measures." But you don't want to make that decision totally.

GAYLENE: I wondered if this wanting to discontinue treatment was selfish on my part because I didn't want to have to cope with the thought of dealing with a very severely handicapped child. And as I did learn to cope with that, I did come to terms with it and then I started wondering about the doctors. And at one point I did say to the doctor, "I've come to terms with where I stand on my selfishness, but I haven't come to terms with you. And have you come to terms with your real feelings about this? I mean is there a selfish desire on your part to do everything you can just to keep this little body breathing so that at the end of three or four months, or whatever it is, you're going to hand me this perhaps severely handicapped child? And you're going to turn around and say, "We did it, we saved another baby, it's going to look really good on our records." And I'm going to be left with this incredible burden. And he said, "Oh no. No, when you leave here you get a lot of support, we never desert you." But you know, realistically you know that you're the parent and that ultimately everything is on your shoulders.

All of these treatments did cause pain to him. You could see him react. At one point I said something to one doctor, something about the pain and he said, "You know, they're so little they don't really feel that much." And then another time, I asked another doctor and he said, "Yes they do feel pain." And I said, "How can you tell?" Because our son couldn't cry because the tube was going through his vocal cord. And he said, "Oh you don't need to hear the cry, you can see their reaction. You can see very clearly that they feel pain." So it would trouble me so much I would go there and I would see all these things happening to him and I used to say to him, "Look I know this hurts, I know you're in pain, but we're letting them do this to you because we hope that in the future it'll give you a chance for a good healthy life, and we're going to do our best to make up for all of this, we're going to make it up to you."

We would talk about it in the car on the way home, and I'd say, "I can't stand what's going on. I can't stand what's happening to his poor little body." Bill would say, "Well that's the way it is now. It's going to get better. It'll be worth it in the long run." But eventually I found that the pain started to erode my optimism. And the more he suffered the closer I was to giving up. Even if he were to be totally healthy, which we knew he wasn't going to be, is putting him through this incredible stuff really going to be worth it in the long run? We were really torn about that.

And then, one day the doctors called us in and said, "Well, it's quite clear now that it's not a matter of whether he's going to survive but the quality of life that he's going to have, because he's doing really well, he is going to survive." You know, half of me sort-of said, "He's going to live, he's going to live." And the other...

The first thing Bill said to the doctors was, "Does that mean now that we don't have the right to say stop treatment any more?" And I think this really shocked them, because they kind of looked at each other and they looked at us, and I know that question caught them off guard because it totally floored me, because up to that point Bill had been the one who was constantly saying, "You know there's life there. We've got to do what we can to save our son's life. We've got to do anything, anything is all right as long as it saves our son's life." And then suddenly he says, "Does that mean we can't stop treatment now?"

BILL: It was quite a memorable meeting that's for sure. I remember up until then thinking: well, if things go wrong or something doesn't work out right, we have the option of ending it there. But now, after this meeting, telling us he's going to live now, so there goes my out... and it was just overwhelming, the larger consequences of it all. I remember talking to the doctors about how far this decision really had gone along, asking could I make the decision later anyway? And they were telling me about the medical review boards, and I can remember reading the paper about other cases in Canada around that time, of people who were fighting doctors for their babies' lives. And it was... it was really quite draining.

GAYLENE: Well, what precipitated this whole thing was that they wanted to do heart surgery on him. And they knew that the way we felt before, we would never have given our okay. And then, with this new dramatic change of things, that yes, he is going to get better, and therefore we feel it's very important that we do as much as we can to maximize his chances for success, that this heart surgery is necessary.

So he had the heart surgery, and he seemed to be rallying very well, except he wasn't putting on weight, and quite suddenly he took a turn for the worse and we could see him beginning to deteriorate very quickly. And that's when... that's when I started getting all kinds of other feelings about what was going on, because all kinds of things would crop up you see. And they would start treating them and before we knew it, it was worse than at the beginning. All kinds of tubes and all kinds of things being done to him, and at him. And I started questioning other procedures and I started saying, "Well, what are the long-term effects of all these x-rays that you're doing?" Then one person would say, "Oh there is no long-term effect." And I would say, "Well I thought that radiation was supposed to be dangerous." I finally asked the one doctor who seemed sympathetic and he said, "Well, we really don't know what the long-term effects are." And I started saying, "Are you doing all this just so that in ten years I can come back to the cancer clinic with this baby?" I started asking again, we're doing all these things for what? For what?

Before we weren't sure, if we stopped treatment, whether we were cheating him of a chance; but at this point he had gotten the chance and things weren't working out anyway, so we felt the decision had been made for us by nature if you like. This is not meant to be, so we can stop all of this fooling around now.

When Bill asked the doctor: do we have any rights now about saying what treatment, about stopping treatment, he said, "Well, that would have to go before a medical ethics committee."

BILL: It seemed harder now, that's for sure, than it was earlier. Now the doctors felt that they had to do everything possible to let him live.

GAYLENE: He got this blood infection and they started this other treatment and I said, "What are we doing here?" It was so clear that he was dying, you could see his body literally deteriorating. He was getting bloated up, obviously from the kidney failure, and you could see this purplish cast which they said was caused from the liver failure, and all of these things were happening, and I remember saying to the one doctor, "You know, what are you doing, why this? " They were doing all these tests that were really painful and they were doing spinal taps and all these other kinds of things that just looked so horrible to me. I said, "Why are you doing all of these tests at this point? We can see he's dying." She said, "We want to find out how he got this blood infection, and we're trying different antibiotics, but none of them seems to be working." And I said, "Hey wait a minute, you know this is really an important thing we have to discuss." And she said, "Well, you know we had a liver specialist in and we had a kidney specialist in." And I said, "Yeah, so you're looking at a liver, he's looking at a kidney and somebody else is looking at blood." But I said, "I'm looking at my baby, I'm looking at this human being, and I'm the only one who can talk for him and what I'm saying to you is stop fooling around with all these tiny little things that are going wrong." They got so enmeshed in this tiny little thing and that tiny little thing, that they lost sight of the whole thing, that there was a real human being here and this real human being was suffering and dying.

Finally, the doctors called us in. And I said, "He's dying isn't he?" And one doctor said, "Well I wouldn't say that." I said, "Well what would you say?" He said, "Well, I would say it's time to consider more invasive treatment." And I said, "Well what did you have in mind?" And he said, "Well we're thinking of dialysis." And I said, "Dialysis, what would that do?" He said, "Well it would relieve the pressure from the kidneys." And I said, "What about the liver? And what about the lungs? What about the brain?" I said, "Is that going to cure his kidney disease, if you do dialysis is it going to cure it?" And he said, "No." And I said, "Well what is it going to do? Why are you going to do all these things?" He said, "Well it might give him a little more time." I said, "A little more time for what? So that you can keep poking him and prodding him and torturing him? Time for what?" I said, "This has just got to stop." The other doctor there finally spoke up and he said, "I agree."

They still said they couldn't remove all of the tubes and things from him, because that still would have to go before the medical ethics committee even though it was so clear that he was dying. How it stopped was that they didn't do the dialysis. They didn't stop treating for the blood infection though. He was still on antibiotics right 'til the end.

He was in a spot in the nursery where everybody could see him, anybody coming in the door would have to see him, even to go and visit other babies. I said, "Could we have a more private spot to be alone with him while he's dying?" The doctor said, "That might be difficult, because the nurses might resent it. They might feel that somehow if we move a baby off that we're giving up on him, and we don't want anybody to think that we're ever giving up." I don't see it as giving up. I don't see it as a failure. His death wasn't a failure, his death was a release. So we put in a request that he be put somewhere more private and that request was honoured, he was put into a private room.

BILL: It was so obvious by this time that there was no other option, that from there 'til the end it was a matter of just trying to make the dying as comfortable as possible.

GAYLENE: We would have really liked to have those tubes out at the end because when we went into see him the last day he had his both arms strapped down on boards, with the IVs and I remember Bill saying to the nurse, "Couldn't we just undo that one arm because he likes to hold our hand with that?" And they said, "No, I'm sorry we can't do that." But they did let us hold him. They wrapped him up and they put him in our arms and he... he just... he struggled and he opened his eyes, and he looked at me, and then he just went totally peaceful.

(Jean André died six weeks after his birth.)

To Hurt and To Heal is distributed by SKY WORKS, 566 Palmerston Ave., Toronto, Ontario, M6G 2P7. (Fax: 416 536-7728)

26

WOMEN'S "CHILDBEARING AGE" AS BIOMEDICAL [RE]CREATION: PRENATAL TESTING AND POSTMENOPAUSAL PREGNANCY

Abby Lippman

Our imminent arrival at the end of the 20th century notwithstanding, women in North America are still evaluated primarily by our reproductive performance and the extent to which we produce babies (Martin, 1990) — babies of certain kinds, I might add.

Aging influences this value in many ways. At the least, some aging is required before a female is able to bear a child; subsequent aging then removes this possibility. But the impact of aging is far more complicated than these biological dynamics. Aging may be a natural process in the life cycle of all women — as well as a lifetime experience we all share — yet it is also, and distinctly, a cultural process whose meaning varies with assumptions about women's roles as producers of babies and with the life/living circumstances of the individual. While the biological and cultural processes may coexist, albeit tensely, they are not co-terminous and this is evident in our colloquial use of such terms as chronological age, mental age, social age and emotional age, as well as in the frequent discordance between them.

"Childbearing age" is another adjectivally-defined period of time in women's lives. As a "natural" biological interval, it comprises those years in her life when a woman has the ability spontaneously to procreate, a time generally taken to be bounded by the beginning and ending of monthly ovulatory cycles: menarche and menopause. As a "social" interval, childbearing age comprises those years in her life when the symbolic, as well as the practical, meaning of motherhood become of great, even determinative, importance in a woman's life. The boundaries of this age reflect social customs and cultural values more than they do biological potentialities. (For instance, do we usually think of a 28-year-old nun as being of childbearing age?) And, more and more, the boundaries are beginning to be products of arbitrary criteria established by geneticists and cemented by medical and social policies.

In this paper I want to explore some contemporary (re)constructions of childbearing age produced by the practices of prenatal diagnosis and postmenopausal obstetrics in North America. Both technologies privilege age as central to the pregnant woman's identity, one making it, or its statistical surrogate, a risk to her childbearing, the other presenting it as a preventable limit on her childbearing interval. I want to consider, too, the (mis)match between women's views of childbearing and aging and these normative (re)constructions.

PRENATAL TESTING

Entry to or eligibility for many activities in North America is often attached to chronological age without consideration of the particularities of an individual that perhaps should condition this entry. These age-linked rules determine, for example, when we can get our first driver's license, when we can vote, when we can receive retirement benefits (Barbec, 1989) and, now, when we receive certain interventions during pregnancy.

Chronological age has been symbolically linked to pregnancy through the evocative (provocative?) notion of "teenage pregnancies" as well as through the long-standing characterization (caricature?) of the "elderly primip."[1] This latter linkage has been fine-tuned recently through the construction of the pregnant woman of "advanced maternal age," the woman whose childbearing is at risk because of the probability she will have a child with a specific genetic disorder, Down syndrome.

It has long been known that the statistical probability of giving birth to a baby with Down syndrome increases dramatically with maternal age. This increase with a woman's age is smooth, albeit exponential, a curve, not a stepladder whose rungs are increasingly widely spaced. Every woman has some numerical chance of having a child with Down syndrome. To determine who in Canada (and elsewhere) will or will not be eligible for prenatal testing to identify fetuses with Down syndrome before they are born, a line is drawn across this continuum. This line separates women at "high" risk from those at "low" risk. It makes some specific number of years since a woman's birth salient and its location is historically and politically contingent.

At present, most biomedical specialists (and those who finance their services) in North America have drawn the line at 35 years. This is the general threshold for access to these tests. Yet, though the notion that risk begins at 35 is generally presented — and certainly seems popularly perceived — as a medical fact, the discontinuity imposed by this (as any) cut-off is by all measures arbitrary. This is apparent when we recall that without any evident changes in women or their biology, the North American minimum age for routine access to testing has dropped during the past 15 years from 40 to 35 years, while 38 years was the minimum age for routine access in France, 36 in England.

Arbitrary or not, however, 35 has already come to be seen as a momentous birthday for the pregnant (white, middle-class) woman and it will only be further reified by the growing tendency of geneticists to combine data from multiple laboratory tests to adjust their birthday-based estimate of an individual woman's numerical chance of having a fetus with Down syndrome. These lab data are conjoined to create a person, the pregnant woman "equivalent-in-her-risk-of-having-a-fetus-with-Down-syndrome-to-a-woman-of-35," the woman "as if" 35. This is the woman for whom all available information suggests that her chance of having a fetus with Down syndrome is equal to or greater than that associated merely with being 35. This is the woman who will be treated, with respect to prenatal diagnosis, and no matter her chronological age, as if she were 35 or over. Accordingly, this (re)construction will not only prematurely age women younger than this whose test results make them "like" an older woman over 35, but rejuvenate those past their 35th birthdays whose tests reduce their initial risk estimates.

This adjustment more-or-less turns the notion of maternal age inside out: whereas maternal age alone had been used until recently to estimate the risk for Down syndrome in the fetus, the risk for Down syndrome calculated from lab data is now used to estimate a woman's "age." This constructed birthday substitutes a technologically-based, statistically-derived surrogate defined solely by a fetal risk for Down syndrome[2] for an elapsed period of real time so that women may now become eligible — or ineligible — for prenatal testing merely by being "as if" over (or under) 35 rather than because they were 35 or over.

In this increasingly popular approach, the derivative of a genetic calculus erases differences between individually identifiable women who have lived very different lengths of time. The 28-year-old and the 42-year-old both disappear only to emerge visibly as (or as not) 35-equivalents. Done to determine eligibility for prenatal diagnosis, the statistically packaged woman is now aged by how "old" others define her to be, and what they define as a "high" risk displaces her self-understanding of age and of risk. Geneticists, rather than her sense of herself or her birth certificate — or her mirror — tell a woman how old she is, with her age mattering only because of the risk at which it places her (fetus).

(Interestingly, a similar process of "aging" appears underway with respect to eligibility for newly begun studies of tamoxifen to prevent breast cancer. Women 60 years and over are automatically eligible for these drug trials, but so, too, will be those "as if" 60, the younger women whose birthdays, family histories, reproductive patterns and so on combine to give them the same statistical probability of breast cancer as the de-contextualized 60-year-old.)

POSTMENOPAUSAL OBSTETRICS AND POSTMENOPAUSAL PREGNANCIES

Let me turn now to postmenopausal pregnancies and their construction of the childbearing interval. If proliferating efforts to lower the age of entry to prenatal diagnosis means being old is getting younger all the time (Hubbard, 1984), postmenopausal obstetrics means being young is getting older all the time — at least for certain groups of women. It also means that women will have to work in still another way at not being old, and at proving it.

Once described as a "notable discontinuit[y]" in a generally continuous process of aging, the "termination of reproductive capacity in women" (Stein, 1985) is being displaced, if not erased, as biomedical researchers create pregnancies in women well beyond menopause. Through the purchase, laboratory fertilization and transfer of eggs from younger women to hormonally-modified older women (e.g., Sauer et al., 1993), physicians now offer to provide what they call "equity" to women whose partners, unlike them, retain the ability to become biological fathers with the passage of chronological time.[3]

Even if we temporarily ignore how this reduces parenthood to biological reproduction, privileging but one component (physiological gestation) in the process of becoming a parent, and one wealthy (heterosexual and likely white) group in the population, this tool alleged to correct the termination of production caused by a woman's age is still troublesome. There is no gender neutrality when it comes to matters of age and aging for men and for women.[4]

Furthermore, and more concretely, postmenopausal pregnancy restructures the duration of childbearing age, removes its contextual grounding, reinforces gendered stereotypes about women and diminishes possibilities for progressive social change. Let me clarify these claims a bit.

Biomedical enthusiasm for postmenopausal pregnancies rests on the implicit assumption that if women, like men, can retain (forever?) their biological capacity to produce a child, the equity between the sexes now impossible because women's physiology is a "natural" barrier to it will be fostered.[5] Moreover, as the fledgling field emerges, postmenopausal obstetrics is being promoted as a humane response to the needs of women who "chose" to postpone childbearing while they pursued education and careers (cf. Rutnam, 1991), an argument similar to that used to explain why women "need" prenatal diagnosis (or infertility treatment) and a reflection of a similar confusion of lack of conception or infertility with childlessness.

However, "need" and "choice" are charged (even manipulative) words, especially when applied to women, their procreation and their health care, and this would seem to be the case here. True, some (privileged) women may postpone pregnancy until their educations are complete or their careers are established. But in a society where privileged white men's traditional unbroken, linear career pathway is taken as the norm to which women are expected to adapt, this delay may not be a real choice. If prevalent expectations about occupational process do not allow for women's physiology, pregnancy at an earlier age (when it is not only possible spontaneously but also means lower risk for fetal chromosome problems) is necessarily precluded. To the extent that "delay" is socially constructed in this way, postmenopausal pregnancy only offers to "resolve" what should not have even been a problem. For were there to be rescheduling of the workplace/workpace for all, rescheduling the women who are working would not be an issue. At best, "equity" given by biomedicine is of a management, not a substantive nature — and likely applicable to women according to race, ability and class distinctions.

The availability of postmenopausal pregnancy puts additional pressure on women to conform to existing gendered norms and to offer it is to favor a high-tech attempt to remove differences between men and women when low-tech (and less hazardous) social policies would remove the unequal consequences that stem from the differences. If women's physiology is at all an "impairment" to equity between the sexes, is it because the natural rhythms of their lives prevent them from spontaneously participating in the conception of a child after the age of 50 years, as biomedical researchers suggest, or because "their physiology" is invoked by others who position women inequitably socially, making it impossible for them to interrupt their paid-working lives to have children at earlier ages.[6] A social "fix" would be far more effective and safer than a medical "fix."

VOICES OF WOMEN

To learn more about how reproductive technologies reconstruct aging and childbearing, we have begun to interview pregnant women in their 30s about these matters. To these women, age is also an issue in being or becoming pregnant and in being a mother. These women also sever the time for childbearing from absolute chronological time, but they do so by situating it in the context of their lives and consider if and when, for example, they will have the time, patience, maturity and energy to accommodate children's needs. A theme in their stories is a notion of "situational" age. They generally appear to hyphenate childbearing with a stage, rather than an age, of life, and try to determine what is the "right" or the "wrong" time or stage to have a baby based on where they think they "are at." Aware of external societal expectations and demands, these (mostly) middle-class white women who have planned their pregnancies want to "be ready" to be parents, and readiness, rather than being directly age-based, depends on such things as one's stamina and physical and mental resources. Others — not they — make a "big deal" about age. To extend the interval in which biological gestation is possible would make no sense to these women. It would likely make what some already see as a large parent-child age difference so great as to "un-ready" them for mothering by precluding the possibility of participating in the long-term growing up of a child. For these women, equity of a different kind applied well before menopause would be far more desirable than that proposed by biomedicine. These women want equal opportunities to have educations, careers and children.

To conclude, let me repeat my claim that North American biomedicine, through prenatal testing and postmenopausal obstetrics, makes the age of a pregnant woman relevant on its terms and in its numbers. It disjoins women's childbearing age from its chronological and biological bases, makes Down syndrome a private problem for an individual family and allows social choices and cultural definitions to shape what is consequently considered an appropriate, if not risk-free, childbearing age. Regarding Down syndrome as removable and the childbearing interval as of unlimited elasticity, biomedicine structures procreation to accord with its qualitative standards and to conform to current societal norms.

Technology is never neutral, and when applied to women it is necessarily gendered in ways reflecting and supporting prevailing attitudes and customs. Prenatal diagnosis and postmenopausal pregnancies both reflect and reinforce the "production of baby" metaphor that dominates much recent biomedical literature about pregnancy, with prenatal diagnosis presented as a tool to monitor production potentially out of control and postmenopausal obstetrics advanced as a tool to reverse age-based cessation of production. They are part of the same process I have been calling the geneticization of reproduction (see Volume One) and become merged in suggestions that we should collect eggs from women when they are young, freeze and then thaw them out later on so that women need not worry about Down syndrome if they wait to have children! They share a view of female aging as a disease-causing agent and both have the potential to constrain possibilities for needed social change. These features, along with their capacity to shape women, children — all of us — and the society in which we live well into the future make these technologies especially problematic.

ACKNOWLEDGMENT

Support for the research from which this paper derives was provided by the Social Sciences and Humanities Research Council of Canada.

REFERENCES

Barbec E.L., "Worries, aging and desires to be younger in a sample of American middle-aged women." *Med Anthropol* 1989,12:117-129.

Hubbard R., "Personal courage is not enough: Some hazards of childbearing in the 1980s," In *Test-tube women*. London: Pandora Press, 1984, pp331-355.

Martin E., "Science and women's bodies: Forms of anthropological knowledge." In *Body/Politics: Women and the discourse of science*. NY: Routledge, 1990, pp 69-82.

McFalls J.A. Jr., "The risks of reproductive impairment in the later years of childbearing." *Annual Rev Sociol* 1990, 16:491-519.

Rindfuss R.R., Bumpass L.L.., "Age and the sociology of fertility: How old is too old?" In *Social demography*, Taueber K.E., Bumpass L.L., Sweet J.A. (eds). NY: Academic Press, 1978, pp 43-56.

Rutnam R., "Is equity enough? Feminist perspectives on health technology assessment policy." *Austral Fem Studies* 1991, 14:47-56.

Sauer M.V., Paulson R.J., LoboR.A. "Pregnancy after age 50: Application of oocyte donation to women after natural menopause." *Lancet* 1993, 341:321-323.

Stein Z.A. "A woman's age: Childbearing and child rearing." *Amer J Epidemiol* 1985, 121(3):327-342.

NOTES

1   "Primip" is an abbreviation for primiparous, a term that means first birth and thus the phrase refers to a woman who will be giving birth for the first time at what physicians consider an "old(er)" age, usually over 30 years.

2   The availability and use of prenatal testing thus create a technologically-based social category of the "older woman" to stand alongside other technologically-based groups such as "teenage drivers" and "young voters" to which people are affiliated whether or not they ever get behind the wheel of a car or cast a ballot.

3   There are many other very troublesome aspects of these "offers" (beyond their race- and class-based assumptions) such as the extent to which they allow the perpetuation of workplace exposures that make pregnancy harder to achieve for certain women, maintain the development of forms of contraception that impair women's "natural" biological fertility and fail to challenge the political and economic systems of North America that encourage later rather than earlier childbearing for some groups of women, but exploring these is beyond the scope of this chapter and they are being dealt with elsewhere.

4   This is apparent when an editorial in a prestigious medical journal, The *Lancet* (6 February 1993), first notes that age is no longer a bar to pregnancy and then asks "is it wise for women in middle and old age to rear young children through to adulthood?" When, we must wonder, was this question asked of older men.

5   It also rests on the assumption that menopause is always and necessarily unwelcome when many women may, in fact, look forward to the relief it provides from menstrual symptoms, from worry about accidental pregnancies and, for those who have been unable or unwilling to become pregnant, from prying questions about why they are not yet pregnant.

6   And, though initiated supposedly for women who have not (yet) had all the children they wanted and who can afford this expensive manipulation, since those who have given birth to the number they wanted may welcome the menstrual freedom of menopause, postmenopausal pregnancy has consequences for all women to the extent that they can be made "responsible" for leaving school or jobs early on to have children. This, in turn, engenders a tone of "blaming the victim" (e.g., McFalls, Jr., 1990) in discussions of women who "choose" to delay childbearing and then, because of biological changes, end up with fewer than were wanted (Rindfass and Bumpass, 1978). Moreover, it poses menopause-timed cessation of childbearing as a choice and thus an area in which pressure to perform can be put on women. And this may be especially so to the extent that it enables family members to put pressure on female relatives to become contract mothers (see chapters by Eichler and Sherwin in this volume).

27

THE ROUTINIZATION OF THE OTHER: ULTRASOUND, WOMEN AND THE FETUS

Lisa M. Mitchell

In only thirty years, the act of gazing upon the fetus within a woman's body has become a routine and expected part of pregnancy for many women in Canada the United States and Europe. In 1957 in Scotland, Ian Donald, or, perhaps, "his" nurse Marjorie Marr, was the first to use ultrasound to create an image of the fetus in utero (Donald, 1980). Today, the conversion of high energy sound waves into an image of a woman's uterus, placenta and moving fetus is widely hailed by obstetricians as the most important "non-invasive" form of prenatal diagnosis. Pregnant women throughout much of Europe, Australia, the United States, as well as Canada, now "routinely" undergo at least one or two ultrasounds (Anderson, 1992; Blondel et al., 1989; Brown and Lumley, 1989 cited in Lumley, 1990; Heringa and Huisjes, 1988; NIH, 1984).

Proponents of ultrasound argue that it is a neutral and passive technology, "a window of unsurpassed clarity into the gravid uterus... capable of providing exquisite detail regarding the fetus and the intrauterine environment" (Pretorius and Mahoney, 1990:1). Medical arguments for the routine use of ultrasound are grounded in the rationale of preventive medicine, economics and individual choice. Routine ultrasound, it is argued, means fewer pre- or post-term babies, fewer "costly" low birth-weight babies, fewer unanticipated complications at childbirth (e.g., placenta previa or breech birth), and the early detection of fetal anomalies so that parents have the "choice" of terminating the pregnancy or preparing for the birth of child with disabilities (Callen, 1988; Pretorius and Mahoney, 1990; Society of Obstetricians and Gynaecologists of Canada, 1981). Medical critics of the routinization of this technology argue that there is still no clear and consistent evidence that ultrasound is safe or that its use in all pregnancies improves maternal or neonatal health or is cost effective (Ewigman, 1989). Routine scans are generally much shorter than the time needed for a detailed search for anomalies and it has been estimated that only about 50 percent of fetal anomalies can be visualised through ultrasound (Toi, 1990).[1]

The routinization of prenatal ultrasound imaging involves not only questions of clinical efficacy and cost-benefit, but social issues of monitoring and control. Authors such as Arney (1982), Oakley (1986), Petchesky (1987; 1990), Rapp (1990) and Rothman (1986;1989) have argued persuasively that reproductive technologies, including ultrasound, are a form of social control, a means of monitoring not only fetal bodies (screening out those which do not conform to "normal") but also women's behaviour (including women's compliance, maternal-fetal "bonding"). Clinicians are not unaware of this aspect of ultrasound. Seeing the fetus through ultrasound is held to reduce women's anxiety (Campbell et al., 1982; Cox et al., 1987; Field et al., 1985; Hyde, 1986; Michelacci et al., 1988; Reading et al., 1988), stimulate their emotional attachment or "bond" with the fetus (Fletcher and Evans, 1983; Garel and Franc, 1980; Kohn et al., 1980; Milne and Rich, 1981; Villeneuve et al., 1988) and encourage compliance with prenatal care (Reading et al., 1982). Ultrasound "windows" are influential in shaping the social relationships of pregnancy, including medicine's claim of authority over the management of pregnancy and the relationship between a pregnant woman and her fetus. As Oakley (1986:155) writes, ultrasound enables physicians "to dispense with mothers as... necessary informants on fetal status and life style." The experiential aspects of pregnancy are obscured and devalued, pregnant women become containers (a "gravid uterus"), backgrounds, the space around a fetus (a "maternal environment") or tissue which may or may not provide a clear ultrasound image.[2] Ultrasound images fix the medical gaze on the fetus, not only as an object of surveillance, diagnosis and therapy but also as a subject, an actor separate from the woman.

Visions of the fetus as the primary obstetrical patient underlie a growing distrust of women to protect the fetus, the rise of "fetal advocates" and an increasing number of court battles over maternal versus fetal "rights" in abortion, "fetal abuse," and decisions about cesarean deliveries (Irwin and Jordan, 1987).

In this paper I draw from the meanings which ultrasound imaging hold for a group of pregnant women in Montreal to examine critically the routine use of this technology.[3] I focus on the significance these women give to the ultrasound image in creating themselves as "mothers" and the fetus as a separate individual. Each of the 49 women was expecting her first child. As are the majority of Canadian women who undergo ultrasound, the women interviewed were at "low risk" for fetal anomalies or complications of pregnancy and childbirth.[4] As is common in Canadian teaching hospitals, each woman had two "routine" prenatal scans (and some had additional "non-routine" ultrasounds).[5] I interviewed each woman on several occasions: before and after her first routine scan, before her second routine scan and post-partum. I also observed their ultrasounds. In this paper I concentrate on the first routine scan which usually occurs at about 18 weeks into the pregnancy.

WOMEN'S EXPECTATIONS ABOUT ULTRASOUND

The women in this study told me that their physicians said little or nothing about ultrasound (except to enquire if they had booked an appointment). Instead, they learned about the procedure, what it would feel like, why it was done and what the image would look like, through conversations with other women and by reading popular guides to pregnancy. None of the women I interviewed were asked if they wanted the ultrasound and their consent was not requested for the procedure, nor did they expect to be asked. Although a woman's consent must be obtained for fetal genetic screening (e.g., amniocentesis, chorionic villus testing), physicians do not have to request a woman's consent for ultrasound. Lippman (1986:442) thus refers to ultrasound as "the first non-voluntary application of prenatal diagnosis." Ultrasound was understood by these women to be routine: it's "another one of those tests they do when you're pregnant." What made this test distinctive and desired was "seeing the baby."

Ultrasound's promise of "seeing the baby" links women to different realms of meaning. First, within current obstetrical thinking, women and fetuses are either at "low risk" or "high risk" for developing problems; there is no state of "no risk." Risk is what justifies the routine widespread use of ultrasound to "catch" fetal anomalies. Quéniart (1987;1992), in her research among pregnant women in Montreal, makes the important point that this "ideology of risk" situates responsibility for the outcome of pregnancy primarily on women and to a lesser degree on physicians and, I would add, sonographers. Unspoken, but assumed, is the belief that "good" mothers do not "take risks" and therefore avail themselves of this technology. Risk is what compels women to come for ultrasound, "just in case." The women I interviewed regarded ultrasound as a way to "reduce the risks" of miscarriage or bearing a child with an anomaly. But thinking about ultrasound in terms of "risks" brought considerable anxiety about the possibility of an anomaly and potential conflicts between maternal altruism and choosing not to bear a child with a disability.[6] Conflicting with their emerging sense of self as "mothers" was the concern spontaneously expressed by about one-half of the 49 women that the ultrasound might harm the fetus or lead to hearing loss, ear infections, cancer, or nervousness in their infants. The risk of harm from the ultrasound was perceived as "small," but, paradoxically, one that had to be taken in order to reduce the risks of fetal anomaly.[7] Several women reassured themselves of ultrasound's safety by reasoning that "everyone has them now" and that doctors "wouldn't be doing ultrasounds if they were dangerous."

Second, "seeing the baby" also refers to women's expectations that they will see "what the baby looks like." Well before the first ultrasound, most of these women had read about fetal development and seen photographs of fetuses in their guides to pregnancy.[8] As they talked to the fetus, imagined its appearance, gender and character, and attempted to "eat better," "rest more" and "take care," women began to create the fetus as an individual and to think about themselves differently, even as mothers. However, prior to the first ultrasound, they talked much more about "being pregnant" than about "having a baby" or about what was inside their bodies. They believe that the ultrasound will allow them to see something — activity, character, family resemblance, gender —

149

which will personalize their baby and, thereby, clarify the identity of the "other." "Seeing the baby," in this sense, refers not only to the cultural meaning of the fetus as a distinctive individual, but also to a woman's relationship with the individual. Hence, the women's comments that through ultrasound they will "get to know," "bond with" and "feel closer" to their baby.

SONOGRAPHERS: "SHOWING THE BABY"[9]

At the hospital where these women had ultrasound, a routine prenatal scan lasts about 15 minutes. During the scan, the sonographer[10] determines the existence of a fetal heartbeat and the position and number of fetuses. She carries out a number of measurements to determine the fetal age, size, development and expected due date. She examines the fetus for any gross physical anomalies and may also note whether it is male or female.

Aside from a few words about the procedure and a brief summary of the findings, relatively little of what sonographers said to these women concerned either technical or diagnostic information. Most of their remarks during a routine ultrasound referred to the anatomy, appearance and activity of the "baby" (the term "fetus" is generally restricted to diagnostic matters). Thus the ultrasound image is often described in terms of the baby's intentional activity ("playing," "swimming," "thinking," "stretching," "resting"), its baby-like appearance ("cute little toes" and "sweet faces") or even its resemblance to other family members. Fetal movement and position were also described as fetal moods, a sign, for example, that the "baby" is "happy," "relaxed," "tired," "shy," or "doesn't like" some aspect of the examination. Occasionally, sonographers interact with the on-screen fetal image, waving "Hello" and giving instructions, words of encouragement or reprimand. They may even touch, stroke and "tickle" the on-screen image or create a voice so the fetus may "speak" to the expectant couple and communicate its "feelings."

Not only is the collection of echoes seen during ultrasound described, talked about and talked to as if it were an individual, a self-acting, conscious and sentient "baby," but the sonographers' accounts also reflect assumptions about normative parental behaviour. The pregnant woman and her partner may be referred to as "Mama" and "Papa." Women who the sonographers feel display evidence of caring about the fetus, that is, interest in the image, concern about fetal health and not too much interest in fetal gender, are called "nice patients." These women tend to receive detailed descriptions of the fetal image. In contrast, less elaborate accounts of the image may be given to women who seem disinterested in the image and more concerned about fetal gender than fetal health. Women who are perceived by the sonographer as overly interested in learning the fetal sex may hear, "Finding out the sex isn't important. The most important thing is that the baby is healthy." Women who admit to smoking during pregnancy may be shown the image of the placenta and told, incorrectly, "we can see the smoke in it." Obese women, told that "it's hard to see," are reminded that their bodies hinder a thorough examination of the fetus.

WOMEN: "SEEING THE BABY"

What do pregnant women say about these fetal images?

When I first looked at it, I couldn't see anything. Emptiness, whiteness. She [the sonographer] *showed me the head, spine, placenta, arms, and the heart. The heart was easy. But if she hadn't said, "Here is the baby," I wouldn't have seen. It was, like, okay, I'll take your word for it.... Now that I've seen it, I have a picture in my mind. To be honest, I didn't have one before. I just couldn't imagine it. And I guess I have a different feeling about it. A better feeling. I feel more relaxed. I know they can't tell me everything about it, but I feel more reassured (Adriana, 26, data and systems clerk).*[11]

To tell you the truth I couldn't see very much.... I saw the outline of the baby's body, the head. The best part was the heart beat, finding something that you could really see. You could see it moving. Other than that it was just kind of the outline, like, of the arm. The body you couldn't really make out, it was just a round clump. I guess the legs were up. I couldn't make out any legs.... I would never have known it was a baby. I would never have recognized anything if it hadn't been pointed out. If I were to look at it again, I doubt I would recognize it (Esther, 27, administrator).

In fact, most women told me that they did not see the fetal shape or outline. They did not recognize what the sonographer was pointing to and saw only the heart, outline of the top of the head, the white line of the fetal femur or the white blocks of the spine. Yet, even if they recall few specifics in the fetal image, most women say they have "seen the baby."

Having "seen the baby" had several meanings. For most women, the ultrasound allows them to re-position themselves in the discourse of fetal risk and normality. Hearing the sonographer say "everything is fine" and seeing the heart beat or fetal movement were met with relief and accepted by most women as evidence that they will give birth to "a normal baby." This evidence can be empowering, at least temporarily, enabling women (especially those with a previous miscarriage) to feel they can publicize the pregnancy by wearing maternity clothes, telling friends and family and making plans for the baby's arrival. The pregnancy is no longer "tentative" (Rothman 1986).

"Seeing the baby" meant more than knowing it was "normal" however. Women used what they saw in ultrasound images and heard from the sonographers to give the fetus a social identity as someone about whom the women knew things such as gender, behaviour, character and family resemblance. Although sonographers at this hospital maintain the first ultrasound is too early to determine fetal sex, women may draw their own conclusions about whether they are having a boy or a girl. In language echoing both the sonographers' comments and gender stereotypes, women explained how they knew it was a boy because the ultrasound fetus was "big," "sturdy" or fast moving, while "delicate," "skinny" and "quiet" ultrasound images signified a girl. Family resemblances in the ultrasound image, comparisons between the fetus and their own or their partner's appearance, character and behaviour are woven into many women's accounts.

> I think the baby will be very calm as opposed to seeing my sister's baby which moved a lot during the ultrasound.... I know now it's gonna have my attitude. It was calm and slow moving. If it was more like my husband, the baby would move a lot more and pace around. I mean, my husband's a great guy, but I'm glad it's gonna have my personality (Marie-Claude, 27, sales clerk, unemployed).

> *The baby's taken on a character that we didn't know before. The fact that she [the sonographer] mentioned the baby was sleeping with its hands over its head. That got to me, because that's exactly how I sleep. So that struck me as being very odd. And the character, the fact that it used its hands a lot. That gave us a kick because I use my hands a lot (Cathy, 33, office manager).*

Fetal movement and the sonographers' descriptions of that movement were also signs of "what the baby's doing in there" and "how it's feeling." Women described this on-screen movement, or lack of it, in a variety of ways: "I saw the baby sleeping," "He was dancing," "I saw my child sitting so peacefully." Sometimes fetal movements were interpreted by women as signs of their baby's character or personality. In words which recall sonographers talking and waving to the fetus, women may describe the movement of the fetal hand as a communicative gesture, saying: "It waved at us" or "It was like the baby said 'Hello' to me."

"BABY'S FIRST PICTURE": ULTRASOUND AS PROOF

In general, routine fetal images are accepted by women as authentic and compelling, as a reliable window through which to observe their baby, and the sonographer's comments as meaningful descriptions of that baby. The image was particularly meaningful as evidence of the "other" and of their own changed identity. Nearly all the women I interviewed talked about the fetal image as a form of proof, saying "Now I know I'm really pregnant!" "Now I know it's real!" or "Now I know there's a baby in there." Having this proof enabled women to talk more confidently about "the baby" and avoid the term "fetus" altogether. They said they felt "different now" about themselves, they "felt like a Mummy" when they saw the fetal image or wanted "to take it easier" or "slower" and to "think more about the baby."

The convincing quality of the ultrasound image stems in part from its pictorial nature since women initially regarded the ultrasound as more compelling evidence of the existence of the fetus than either a hormonal pregnancy test or hearing the fetal heartbeat. In comparison to the technologically derived evidence of ultrasound, a woman's own bodily sensations and perceptions were suspect.

It's not my imagination. There really is a baby in there. I'm not just getting fat (Jennifer, 31, social services worker).

Seeing the baby meant that it's really there. I'm not imagining things. It's been nearly four months and you can't really see any results. Yes, I'm nauseated and have sore breasts. I'm tired and my stomach is sticking out, but seeing an image of the child, it's reality (Michelle, 27, communications analyst).

The routine ultrasound has become a public ritual in which spouses, family members and sonographers as well as, women, witness the baby and display their relationship to it. The copy of the fetal image received after the scan extends this ritual outside of the clinical context. Women often displayed the fetal ultrasound image in their homes, on the refrigerator, at their bedside or in an album or frame as "Baby's First Picture." Foreshadowing school photos of their children, several men put the image in their wallets or on their desk at work. The symbolic value of the image is so great that even though many could not identify anything in the image, women and men showed it to friends, family members and workmates as "a picture of my baby."

This procedure is so widely a part of the popular understanding of pregnancy and its images so familiar that they are taken for granted as neutral or unconstructed recordings of the fetus. Women equated the ultrasound with a "camera" or a "video" and the resulting image as a "photo." But for some women, this "window" onto the fetus intruded onto their distinctive bodily relationship with the fetus. Since the first routine scan is done at about 16 to 20 weeks gestation, women may see the fetus move before they feel that movement. Seeing this movement prior to quickening reinforced their belief that ultrasound provided authoritative and distinctive information, but for some women it was unsettling.

It was like it [the fetus] moved for her [the sonographer], but not for me (Christina, 25, secretary).

It was neat and all that, you know, to see the baby moving. But, I don't know, I guess I thought the mother was supposed to feel it. Like that's when you know it's there (Tina, 28, social services worker).

By the second routine scan, rationalized by clinicians as a means of screening for anomalies and delays in fetal growth and potential complications of childbirth, women regarded the ultrasound screen as much less rich with information about the fetus. Aside from those who were told whether they were having a boy or girl, only a few women used the second fetal image to further construct the social identity of the fetus. By this point in the pregnancy, nearly all the women regarded fetal movements, felt directly rather than seen through ultrasound, as meaningful signs of fetal health, sentience, character, emotion and behaviour. By post-partum, the distinctiveness and the reliability of ultrasound's vision erode further, as women expressed disappointment and frustration with ultrasound's failure to accurately predict fetal size, long and difficult labours or cesarean deliveries.

CONCLUSION

The act of gazing past the pregnant women at an indistinct collection of echoes which are referred to as the "baby" has become a routine part of pregnancy in much of Canada. The routinization of ultrasound fetal imaging has occurred with virtually no understanding or questioning of the implications of this technology for women's experiences of pregnancy, for the medical management of pregnancy or for the meanings which "fetus," "baby," "mother" and "pregnant woman" hold for physicians, women, men, indeed for any of us. Based on my research, I believe that the process by which women having routine scans define both themselves and the fetus is now entangled with ultrasound. Among these Montreal women, "seeing the baby" was a ritualized, technological and public quickening, a sign not just of life but of redefined selves and emerging others. Women's bodily sensations, imagined babies and the generalized fetuses in their pregnancy guide books became more sharply focussed into a distinctive individual, a social actor with an identity, character and rights. That spotlight on the "baby" cast new meanings on a woman's sense of herself. Women's willingness to define themselves not just as pregnant but as "having a baby" or to do so publicly drew heavily from the interpretation of a "normal" ultrasound. Their sense of "being a mother" drew upon ultrasound's perceived ability to reduce risks, help them "bond with their baby" and offer proof to others that they had done so.

Ultrasound does not make fetuses into babies or women into mothers; these social transformations in meaning are far more complex. Nevertheless, what ultrasound images "say" about the fetus and about the pregnant woman are subject to multiple interpretations and, hence, (mis)uses. Some troubling examples have surfaced. *The Silent Scream,* the film purporting to use ultrasound images of a fetus during an abortion, is perhaps only the most (in)famous (Petchesky, 1987). Lippman (1986:442) mentions that some American lawmakers wanted mandatory viewing of ultrasound fetal images as an attempt to dissuade pregnant women from having an abortion. The commercial use of ultrasound solely to determine the sex of the fetus drew the attention of the Canadian media briefly in 1990.[12] For the most part, however, ultrasound fetal images are not regarded as ethically or socially problematic. The use of an ultrasound fetal image to advertise what is widely regarded as a "safe" brand of car highlights the extent to which these images have become both popularized and synonymous with responsible, caring behaviour toward the fetus.[13] My own research suggests that normative expectations about maternal behaviour are part of how ultrasound is made meaningful for both women and sonographers. Statements in the clinical literature that ultrasound may encourage maternal-fetal bonding and improve compliance with prenatal care raise the troubling spectre that routine scans may be used to "correct" women's behaviour during pregnancy (Lippman, 1986:442). Particularly worrisome is the possibility that if clinical trials do not show clear and consistent benefits to maternal or neonatal health as occurred in a recently published study (Ewigman et al, 1993; Lefevre et al, 1993), then so-called "psychological benefits," the ability of ultrasound to influence maternal behaviour, and women's expectations to have ultrasound will be applied increasingly to justify the routine use of this technology (Acheson and Mitchell, 1994).

REFERENCES

Acheson, Louise and Lisa M. Mitchell, "The routine antenatal diagnostic imaging with ultrasound study: The challenge to practice evidence-based obstetrics" *Archives of Family Medicine*, 1993 (Dec).

American College of Obstetricians and Gynecologists, *Ultrasound in Pregnancy. Technical Bulletin* No. 116. Washington, D.C.: American College of Obstetricians and Gynecologists1988.

Anderson, G.M., *An Analysis of Temporal and Regional Trends in the Use of Prenatal Ultrasonography*. Ottawa: Royal Commission on New Reproductive Technologies 1992.

Arney, William R., *Power and the Profession of Obstetrics*. Chicago: The Univ. of Chicago Press 1982.

Beech, Beverly, et al., *A Commentary on the Report of the Royal College of Obstetricians and Gynaecologists Working Party on Routine Ultrasound Examination in Pregnancy*. London: Association for Improvements in the Maternity Services 1985.

Blondel, Beatrice, et al., "The use of ultrasound examinations, intrapartum fetal heart rate monitoring and beta-mimetic drugs in France." *British Journal of Obstetrics and Gynaecology*. 96 Jan1989:44-51.

Callen, Peter, *Ultrasonography in Obstetrics and Gynecology*. Philadelphia: W.B. Saunders 1988.

Campbell, S., et al., "Ultrasound scanning in pregnancy: the short-term psychological effects of early real-time scans." *Journal of Psychosomatic Obstetrics and Gynaecology* 1982 1-2:57-61.

Corporation professionnelle des médecins du Québec, *The Practice of Obstetrics: Patient Care during Pregnancy, Obstetrical Echography*. Montréal: CPMQ 1987, *Nine Months for Life*. Montréal: CPMQ 1990

Cox, David, et al., "The psychological impact of diagnostic ultrasound." *Obstetrics and Gynecology* 1987.

Donald, Ian, *Medical sonar — the first 25 years. In Recent Advances in Ultrasound Diagnosis*, Vol II. Asim Kurjak, ed. Pp. 4-20. Amsterdam: Excerpta Medical Publishers 1980.

Eisenberg, Arlene, et al., *What to Expect When you are Expecting* New York: Workman 1988.

Ewigman, Bernard, "Should ultrasound be used routinely during pregnancy? An opposing view." *Journal of Family Practice* 1989 29(6):660-664.

Ewigman, B.G., J.P. Crane, .F.O. Frigoletto et al. "Effect of prenatal ultrasound screening on perinatal outcome." *New England Journal of Medicine*, 1993, 329: 821-827.

Field, Tiffany, et al., "Effects of ultrasound feedback on pregnancy anxiety, fetal activity, and neonatal outcome." *Obstetrics and Gynecology* 1985 66(4):525-528.

Fletcher, John and Mark Evans, "Maternal bonding in early fetal ultrasound examinations." *New England Journal of Medicine* 1983 308(7):392-393.

Garel, M. and M. Franc, "Réactions des femmes à l'échographie obstétricale." *Journal of Gynaecology, Obstetrics, Biology and Reproduction* 1980 9:347-354.

Harrison, Michael, "Unborn: historical perspective of the fetus as a patient." *The Pharos* Winter 1982..

Heringa, M. and H.J. Huisjes, "Prenatal screening: current policy in EC countries." *European Journal of Obstetrics and Gynecology* 1988 28 (Supplement):7-52.

Hyde, Beverley, "An interview study of pregnant women's attitudes to ultrasound scanning." *Social Science and Medicine* 1986 22(5):587-592.

Irwin, Susan and Brigitte Jordan, "Knowledge, practice, and power: court-ordered cesarean sections." *Medical Anthropology Quarterly* 1987 (n.s.) 1(3):319-334.

Jackson, R. , "The use of ultrasound in obstetrics." *Irish Medical Journal* 1985 78(6):149-150

Kitzinger, Sheila, *The Complete Book of Pregnancy and Childbirth*. New York: Alfred K. Knopf 1989.

Kohn, C.L. et al., "Gravidas' responses to realtime ultrasound fetal image." *Journal of Obstetrics, Gynecology and Neonatology in Nursing* 1980 9:77-80.

The Lancet, "Diagnostic ultrasound in pregnancy: WHO view on routine screening" [editorial]. *The Lancet* (Aug 11 1984 :361.

"Minister's warning about routine use of ultrasound in pregnancy" [editorial]. *The Lancet* (Oct 27 1984):995.

Layne, Linda L., "Of fetuses and angels: fragmentation and integration in narratives of pregnancy loss. Knowledge and Society," *The Anthropology of Science and Technology.*1992 9:29-58.

Lefevre, ML, R.P. Bain, B.G. Ewigman et al. "A randomized trial of prenatal ultrasonographic screening: impact on maternal management and outcome. *Amer. J. Obstet. and Gynecology* 1993 169: 483-489

Lippman, Abby, "Access to prenatal screening services: who decides." *Canadian Journal of Women and the Law* 1986 1(2):434-445.

Lumley, Judith, "Through a glass darkly: ultrasound and prenatal bonding." *Birth* 1990 17(4):214-217.

Michelacci, L., et al., "Psychological reactions to ultrasound." *Psychother Psychosom* 1988 50:1-4.

Milne, L.and O. Rich, "Cognitive and affective aspects of the responses of pregnant women to sonography." *Maternal-Child Nursing Journal* 1981 10:15-39.

Mitchell, Lisa M., *Making Babies: The Cultural Construction of the Fetus and Routine Ultrasound Imaging in Montréal, Canada.* Unpublished 1993 PhD Dissertation, Anthropology, Case Western Reserve University, Cleveland, Ohio.

National Institutes of Health, "The use of diagnostic ultrasound imaging in pregnancy." NIH Consensus Development Conference Statement (Feb. 6-8, 1984). *Journal of Nurse-Midwifery* 1984 29(4):235-239.

Oakley, Ann, *The Captured Womb: A History of the Medical Care of Pregnant Women.* Oxford: Basil Blackwell 1986.

Petchesky, R., "Fetal images: the power of visual culture in the politics of reproduction." In *Reproductive Technologies: Gender, Motherhood and Medicine.* M. Stanworth, ed. Pp.57-80. Minneapolis: University of Minnesota Press 1987.

Abortion and Woman's Choice: The State, Sexuality, and Reproductive Freedom, revised edition. Boston: Northeastern University Press 1990.

Pretorius, Jack Dolores and Barry S. Mahoney, *The role of obstetrical ultrasound.* In *Diagnostic Ultrasound of Fetal Anomalies: Text and Atlas.* David Nyberg et al., eds. Pp.1-20. Chicago Year Book Medical Publishers 1990.

Quéniart, Anne, "La technologie: un réponse à l'insécurité des femmes?" In *Accoucher Autrement.* Francine Saillant et Michel O'Neill, eds. Pp. 213-235. Montréal: Éditions Saint-Martin 1987.

Risky business: medical definitions of pregnancy. In *The Anatomy of Gender.* D. Currie and V. Raoul, eds. Pp. 161-174. Ottawa: Carleton University Press 1992.

Rapp, Rayna, "The power of 'positive' diagnosis: medical and maternal discourse on amniocentesis." In Karen Michaelson et al, *Childbirth in America: Anthropological Perspectives.* Pp. 103-116. South Hadley, Mass: Bergin and Garvey Pub 1988.

"Constructing amniocentesis: maternal and medical discourses." In *Uncertain Terms: Negotiating Gender in American Culture.* Faye Ginsburg and Anna Lowenhaupt Tsing, ed. Pp. 28-42. Boston: Beacon Press 1990.

Reading, Anthony, et al., "Health beliefs and health care behaviour in pregnancy." *Psychological Medicine* 1982 12:379-383.

"A controlled, prospective evaluation of the acceptability of ultrasound in prenatal care." *Journal of Psychosomatic Obstetrics and Gynecology* 1988 8:191-198.

Reece, E. Albert, et al., "The safety of obstetric ultrasonography: concern for the fetus." *Obstetrics and Gynecology* 1990 76:139-146.

Rothman, Barbara Katz, *The Tentative Pregnancy: Prenatal Diagnosis and the Future of Motherhood*. New York: Viking Penguin 1986.

Reinventing Motherhood: Ideology and Technology in a Patriarchial Society. New York: W.W.Norton 1989.

Society of Obstetricians and Gynaecologists of Canada, "Guidelines for the use of ultrasound in obstetrics and gynecology." *Bulletin of the Society of Obstetricians and Gynaecologists of Canada* 1981.

Stabile, Carol A., "Shooting the mother: fetal photography and the politics of disappearance." *Camera Obscura* 1992 28:178-205.

Taylor, Janelle, "The public foetus and the family car: From abortion politics to a Volvo advertisement." *Public Culture* 1992 4(2): 67-80.

Toi, A., "Update in ultrasound: fetal diagnosis." *The Canadian Journal of Ob/Gyn* Dec 1990: 125-129.

Youngblood, James, "Should ultrasound be used routinely during pregnancy? An affirmative view." *Journal of Family Practice* 1989 29(6):657-660.

Villeneuve, Claude, et al., "Psychological aspects of ultrasound imaging during pregnancy." *Canadian Journal of Psychiatry* 1988 33:530-535.

NOTES

1   Routine prenatal ultrasound has been reviewed by numerous national and international bodies. Most, but not all, concluded that routine fetal imaging was not warranted based on the evidence concerning its safety and clinical benefit. See, for example, Beech et al. (1985), Jackson (1985), NIH (1984), and *The Lancet* (1984a,b) and, for discussions of clinical benefits of ultrasound, Ewigman (1989), Reece (1990) and Youngblood (1989). In their published guidelines for ultrasound, neither the American College of Obstetricians and Gynecologists (1988) nor the Society of Obstetricians and Gynaecologists in Canada (1981) endorse routine scans. "The Corporation professionnelle des médecins du Québec [says it] has no objection to ultrasonographic screening between the 16th and 20th weeks of pregnancy, even in a woman whose pregnancy appears to be evolving normally" (CPMQ 1987:24).

2   See Petchesky (1990) and Stabile (1992) for two excellent analyses of the obscuring of women in fetal images.

3   The material for this paper comes from a larger study in which I examined how ultrasound's echoes become meaningful as representations of fetal selves among pregnant women and sonographers at a hospital in Montreal. In addition to interviews with pregnant women and observations of their ultrasound, the fieldwork included fifteen months (1989-1991) of observations of ultrasound fetal imaging and multiple interviews with sonographers. My thanks to these sonographers and to the other women and men who participated in this research. The research was funded by a Wenner-

Gren Foundation Predoctoral Research Grant. The studies leading up to the research were funded by a Medical Research Council of Canada International Youth Year Special Studentship.

4   Given the space restraints of this paper, I have not discussed the diversity of meanings which women of different cultural and social positions give to pregnancy, the fetus and ultrasound images. In brief, the conventional Canadian categories of "anglophone," "francophone" and "allophone" (maternal language is neither English nor French) correspond roughly to 60 percent, 20 percent and 20 percent of the women I interviewed. Most were born and raised in Montreal, all were between 22 and 33 years of age and living with a male partner. About one-third of the women had previous pregnancies which ended in miscarriage or abortion.

5   I should clarify that I use the term "routine" at the same time that I contest the need for these scans in all pregnancies. I use the term "non-routine" to refer to those ultrasounds done in addition to the routine "16 week" and "32 week" scans. About one-third of the women had at least one additional scan for a variety of reasons including vaginal bleeding, suspected smaller than average or larger than average fetal size, confirmation of fetal position, follow-up to possible fetal anomaly. About 20 percent of the women underwent at least four ultrasounds during their pregnancy.

6   For this issue in amniocentesis screening see Rapp (1988).

7   Quéniart (1992:167) made the same finding in talking with pregnant women in Montreal about amniocentesis. She writes that, "women feel the need for reassurance at all costs even if it means — and herein is... [a] paradox — taking risks."

8   There were a variety of guides to pregnancy read by the women. Among the more common titles were *What to Expect When You're Expecting* (Eisenberg et al., 1988), *The Complete Book of Pregnancy and Childbirth* (Kitzinger, 1989), *Nine Months for Life* (Corporation professionnelle des médecins du Québec 1990).

9   Elsewhere I have analyzed in detail sonographers' interpretations of the fetal image, what they refer to as "showing the baby" (Mitchell, 1993). What follows here is only a brief summary.

10 In Canada, prenatal ultrasound is provided in a variety of settings, including hospital departments of radiology, obstetrics, and maternal-fetal medicine, in private clinics and in physicians' offices. The scans may be conducted by obstetricians, radiologists and residents in obstetrics and radiology. The routinization of obstetrical ultrasound is paralleled by the increasing numbers of scans carried out by "technicians," rather than physicians. Not insignificantly, most of these technicians are women and their skills are much less costly than those of physicians.

11 I have used pseudonyms for the women and generalized their occupations to avoid disclosing their identities.

12 In the case I am referring to, sex determination by ultrasound was advertised in South Asian communities in British Colombia by a physician near the border in the United States ("As it Happens," CBC radio, Friday Sept 21, 1990). The issue of how widely ultrasounds for sex selection may be available to or requested by women throughout Canada was overshadowed by discussions about sexism in "cultural communities" and the commercial use of reproductive technology.

13 See Taylor's (1992) analysis of the fetal image in this Volvo advertisement.

28

INFORMED CONSENT AND THE PREGNANT WOMAN

Karen Capen

TECHNOLOGIES IN PREGNANCY HEALTH CARE

Physicians, today, have many new technologies available with which to "treat" pregnancy. Some of these new "tools" involve prenatal testing, a practice that has become routine in the past few years. Some of these tests are more "high tech" than others; some tests are also more invasive (and therefore risky to both pregnant woman and fetus). These tests, one of which is ultrasound, have also dramatically shifted the focus of a woman's prenatal care from her own health to that of the fetus.

There are a range of ethical and legal requirements associated with medical care and treatment, one of which is that a patient be adequately informed about diagnostic and therapeutic procedures before they are undertaken. Obtaining valid consent before carrying out any prenatal testing is an example of how this principle should be acted on in standard obstetric practice. It is considered to be an elementary obligation of the physician to the patient.

THE REQUIREMENT OF INFORMED CONSENT

The content of the principle of informed consent, applied to the use of ultrasound in pregnancy, includes several connected issues: the competence of the pregnant woman, her health-related knowledge, her ability to ask questions, the information given to her by her physician and the voluntariness of her decision-making or choice.[1] In the case of a pregnant woman, once a second-trimester ultrasound test has been conducted as part of the routine package of prenatal care, her "choices"[2] if any questionable finding occurs, are that she proceed to have other "confirmatory" tests, that she continue the pregnancy and have a possibly "defective" baby or that she terminate the pregnancy.

Although few women realize it, one of the issues surrounding the routine use of these tests is that none of them, singly or in combination, can establish without any doubt that the development of the fetus is proceeding normally. Even after the baby is born, there is still no way of immediately detecting some genetic or developmental conditions.[3]

Informed consent is critical in pregnancy for a number of reasons. The physician's duty of disclosure today is no longer determined by the information a careful physician might give a patient in similar circumstances. The information provided to a pregnant woman during her prenatal care must now include the information a reasonable woman (in the place of the patient) might want to hear. This means the physician must explain the testing process, provide all information about material or probable risks and identify the range of possible outcomes of the proposed tests a reasonable woman in the pregnant woman's place would want to consider before agreeing to proceed.[4]

GUIDELINES FOR PHYSICIANS

A variety of medical associations and provincial regulating bodies that provide practice-related services to physicians have developed guidelines to assist physicians in meeting the legal standard of medical disclosure, the information component of the informed consent process. However, these requirements for informed consent often operate within the physician/patient relationship in a way that puts the pregnant woman at a disadvantage. This becomes particularly apparent when the complex relationship between a physician and patient is examined.

THE PHYSICIAN/PATIENT RELATIONSHIP

TYPES OF RELATIONSHIPS

The concept of informed consent has emerged from a critical examination of the physician/patient relationship as people search for assurances of safety in an area where the interpretation of technical information places much power in the hands of medical professionals. In studies undertaken in the past two decades in response to struggles arising from the increased attention given to patient autonomy in medical decision-making, a range of dynamics has been identified.

Four particular types of physician/patient relationship have been described:

1. The paternalistic (sometimes called priestly) type of relationship, in which the physician is an authority figure making decisions and providing patient care seen by the physician to be in that patient's best interest;

2. The informative (scientific and consumer-oriented) type, in which the physician provides the patient with diagnostic information and treatment options so that the patient can select the medical care he or she wants;

3. The interpretive type (fiduciary in nature), in which the purpose of the interaction is for physicians to determine each patient's values and needs, in order to help the patient select the most suitable medical interventions; and

4. The deliberative (or collegial) style, in which the physician assists the patient in identifying and choosing the best general approach to his or her health care, including prevention and treatment.

It is the informative model that most specifically suits the informed consent standard. But even though this standard is considered to be more patient-based than it was initially, it is still an unrealistic one given the generally acknowledged power discrepancy between the physician and the pregnant woman patient.[5]

THE FIDUCIARY NATURE OF THE RELATIONSHIP

Some physicians educated today in a humanities-oriented program are likely to operate within the deliberative model. Others with a strong attachment to a science-based professional identity are more associated with the informative model. The law has recently added to this range of dynamics by defining the physician/patient relationship as a fiduciary one.[6] As part of the legal duty that a physician has to inform the patient, it is now generally held that there are also special duties of care and trustworthiness. This means that the physician is bound by a positive obligation to ensure that the patient understands more fully the nature of the procedures and treatment that are to be provided (as in the "interpretive" model).

1. Information on Benefits, Risks and Alternatives

The amount of information that will be considered sufficient within the legal concept of the fiduciary physician/patient relationship must be assessed in the context of the specific relationship. The law also requires a higher standard of disclosure for non-therapeutic procedures than for therapeutic ones.[7] This means that the physician and patient must determine whether the care needed is therapeutic or non-therapeutic in nature. In the case of prenatal care and the routine use of ultrasound, this is a particularly controversial issue. There is concern that some of the procedures that have come to be provided routinely during the prenatal care visits of a pregnant woman with her physician have unproven benefits and may be more experimental than therapeutic. (One example of this is a recent study of childbirth procedures that suggested that routine use of episiotomies, one of the most common surgical procedures in Canada and the U.S., is usually unnecessary and, except for special circumstances [i.e., when the fetus is in distress or, rarely, when the woman cannot push], may do more harm to women than good.[8])

As part of the physician's duty to inform his or her patient, it is also important, with the routine use of ultrasound, to consider what benefits this test provides, and for whom. In the kind of health care system we have today, an implicit recommendation by a medical specialist carries a great deal of weight. In providing information to a pregnant woman, the physician must explain, to adequately fulfil this duty to inform, that an "abnormal" ultrasound will likely require further genetic assessment, and that one alternative she may wish to consider if further tests indicate a genetic or physiological "defect" is termination of the pregnancy. (This is the abortion we have come to recognize as "indicated for medical reasons" or "for the health of the mother.")

2. Routine Testing in Pregnancy

When a relatively non-invasive test such as ultrasound becomes a routine part of prenatal care, it is easy to forget that the implications of its use go far beyond how it is often presented. There is considerable social pressure on the pregnant woman (even if unstated) to consent to the procedures her physician suggests because she fears that the relationship will be damaged if she does not. A test represents attention at a time when many woman equate such attention with care.

Also, because prenatal visits usually occur on a monthly basis, each visit represents an incremental stage of the relationship with new information arising each time. Informed consent under such circumstances is difficult because the cumulative meaning to the woman patient of all the visits during the continuum of prenatal and childbirth care is obscured, thereby diminishing her role in the whole reproductive process. This occurs because the visits are scheduled on a routine basis, placing emphasis on fetal testing and making the patient less visible.

3. Multiple Obligations of Physicians

Another factor to consider is that the obligations of the physician in the physician/patient relationship co-exist with other professional responsibilities of the physician. In our health-care system, the physician also has significant obligations to others, including health-care institutions, medical facilities, and education and research activities.

The emphasis today, given our understanding of the disadvantage of women in the physician/patient relationship, has shifted from the physician's obligation to disclose information (the "informative" type of relationship) to the quality of the patient's understanding and consent. The physician's duty is carefully weighed, partly because of legal concerns. It is unclear as to how the process of informed consent can be shaped to truly meet a standard that respects the interests and autonomy of women given institutional concerns regarding the professionals' capacity to comply. An adequate standard as far as women patients are concerned is seen to be too onerous on the physician because truly informed consent requires more discussion and disclosure than the physician and health-care system can bear. (It may be asked, however, if the system can bear *not* attending to this issue. It is this human dimension, the interaction between physician and woman patient during her pregnancy, which introduces the "quality" aspect into prenatal care.)

DISADVANTAGES FOR WOMEN
THE SOCIAL POWER OF THE MEDICAL PROFESSION

First of all, it is useful to examine some of the underlying social conditions that affect the nature of the physician/pregnant woman patient relationship. During the nineteenth century, medicine as a profession became institutionalized at a time when scientific knowledge was widely becoming associated with "progress." One of the important developments at this time was the increased interest of the medical profession in women's bodies in general, and in women's reproductive processes in particular. The so-called "natural" processes of conception, pregnancy and childbirth came to be seen as "dysfunctional," thus requiring special medical attention.

This emphasis on the scientific approach is considered by some women to be consistent with the general male hegemony in our society, and also to reflect the state's assumption of power over women's lives.[9] According to this analysis, women are not seen by society to be in control of their sexuality and reproductive processes, and coming to believe this, women themselves then turn to those professionals with medical expertise to determine what is best for them. Human reproduction is thus transformed into a variety of specialized medical tests, procedures and treatments in order to secure the safe "delivery" of a perfect baby, rather than to assist in the birth of a woman's child. The shifting of emphasis and responsibility from the pregnant woman to the physician and his or her use of technology is subtle but meaningful in terms of the power imbalance.

GENERAL ATTITUDES TO NEW TECHNOLOGIES

A second reason for the pregnant woman's disadvantage in her relationship with her physician concerns general attitudes in our society to new developments in medical science and technology. For example, a prenatal test such as ultrasound is seen to be an advancement as far as quality medical care is concerned, and once such a test is perceived to be reasonably safe, there is often wide support for its being put to use.[10]

CONSENT AS LIABILITY PROTECTION

A physician, under such circumstances, may feel compelled to use prenatal testing as protection against a possible malpractice suit in the event a particular condition is left undiagnosed until birth. Even if the pregnant woman is offered the option of refusing testing (as suggested in certain guidelines), the tendency will likely be for her to accept the "routine" care that is recommended by the medical professional. This is understandable, given that the alternative for any woman is the extended period of uncertainty associated with pregnancy, even if the information provided by the test is not necessarily relevant or entirely accurate.

Informed consent, and even the validity of any tacit consent, is, in this social context, and under the current definitions and guidelines, a medical and legal fiction.[11] The consent obtained under these circumstances should have little weight. The consent process between a pregnant woman and her physician also requires the ability to form and express an informed dissent to procedures that make assumptions about that particular woman's needs and values. Legitimate consent implies that there will be opportunities to question and even disagree.

TOWARD REAL PARTICIPATION IN PREGNANCY CARE

The question then is: how can prenatal and childbirth care be managed by a pregnant woman in order to ensure that the underlying disadvantages for the woman patient in the physician/patient relationship (gender socialization and professional status[12]) do not prevent her from real participation in the decisions affecting that care. Some possible approaches:[13]

1. A re-emphasis on the woman as the patient (instead of the fetus) in the physician/patient relationship in order to assist the pregnant woman in becoming more active, participatory and responsible;

2. A shift from the "medicalization" of prenatal care in order to place less emphasis on the physical development of the fetus and to focus more on the pregnant woman's social and psychological needs;

3. An acceptance of the special nature of consent during pregnancy and childbirth care so that the process is treated as a continuum, and any deficiencies in the consent obtained, including implied consent, are avoided.

4. The acknowledgment of medical uncertainty regarding the usefulness and even safety of some of the procedures and treatments at the outset of the prenatal care;

5. The creation of a special physician/patient relationship in which consent is seen as a process during which the pregnant woman's questions are encouraged and in which she is given time to reflect on the information provided, both in terms of its adequacy and its attention to her particular needs.

NOTES

1   See *Consent to Medical Care (Protection of Life Series)*, A Study Paper prepared for the Law Reform Commission of Canada, Margaret A. Somerville, 1980. In Chapter II, "The Doctrine of 'Informed' Consent," p.11, Prof. Somerville identifies three main areas: capacity or competence, information or knowledge, and volition. These elements of the process presuppose two equally powerful, autonomous individuals in the physician/patient context.

2   Barbara Katz Rothman has written extensively on the underlying assumptions that exist when we use the term "choice" in any discussion of the new reproductive technologies. See, for example, *Recreating Motherhood: Ideology and Technology in a Patriarchal Society*, New York: W.W. Norton & Company, 1989, p.62.

3   A February 1987 brochure entitled "The Practice of Obstetrics: Patient Care during Pregnancy, Obstetrical Echography" published by the Corporation professionnelle des medecins du Quebec, states: "The popularity of obstetrical echography (ultrasound) derives not only from the valuable diagnostic information it provides but also from its established innocuity.... It is undoubtedly this apparent innocuity...which explains why no body, association or committee has to date expressed any objection to the use of ultrasound in pregnancy if a medical indication for it is considered to exist. At the same time, every group which has studied the safety of ultrasound has insisted on a policy of prudence and has recommended the continuation of research."

Also in 1987, in an article in a Society of Obstetricians and Gynecologists publication called *The Bulletin* (July/August, 1987, p.19) one physician, Dr. Carl A. Nimrod, was quoted as follows: "I am unaware of Canadian studies which prospectively address the issues of routine ultrasound in obstetrics. At least 85 percent of the population will do well in spite of us, therefore one is hardpressed to justify the diagnostic tool which might be considered unnecessary. However, if we look at the other side of the coin, ultrasound does provide a window to the fetus. One must agree that we are seeing through a glass darkly and sometimes the limited vision can cause more harm than good."

4   Supreme Court of Canada cases Hopp v. Lepp [1980] 2 SCR 192, and Reibl v. Hughes [1980] 2 SCR 880 established a new standard of legal disclosure, which requires more attention be given by physicians to pre-procedure or pre-treatment discussions with their patients.

5   The models described here are based on the analysis by Robert M. Veatch in *A Theory of Medical Ethics*, New York: Basic Books Inc. Publishers, 1981, and expanded on in an article, "Four Models of the Physician/Patient Relationship," by E.J. Emanuel and L.L. Emanuel published in *JAMA*, April 22/29, 1992, Volume 267, Number 16, p.2221-2226.

6   McInerney v. MacDonald, [1992] 2 SCR 138.

7   White v. Turner (1981), 31 O.R. (2nd) 773, 15 C.C.L.T. 81, 120 D.L.R. (3rd) 269, affirmed 20 C.C.L.T. xxii (C.A.)

8   *Globe and Mail*, July 7, 1992, "Childbirth procedure questioned," page A1, by Paul Taylor.

9   See, for example, Catharine A. MacKinnon, *Toward a Feminist Theory of the State*, Cambridge, Mass.: Harvard University Press, 1989.

10 Stephen Toulmin makes this point in an essay entitled "Technological Progress and Social Policy," published in *Medical Innovation and Bad Outcomes: Legal, Social and Ethical Responses*, ed. Mark Siegler, Michigan: Health Administration Press, 1987.

11 For further discussion of this point, see "Informed Consent Does Not Mean Rational Consent," by Jon F. Merz and Baruch Fischhoff, *The Journal of Legal Medicine*, 1990, Volume 11, p.321-350.

12 The point here is that there is both the professional status issue and the issue that even physicians who are women have been socialized in their professional training according to male educational standards. So there is actually a double gender socialization issue: that of women generally, and the more subtle professional education one as well.

13 A reading of Susan Sherwin's *No Longer Patient: Feminist Ethics and Health Care* (Philadelphia: Temple University Press, 1992), provided a strong basis for this discussion of possible improvements to the physician/pregnant woman patient relationship.

29

STATE INTERVENTION IN PREGNANCY

Ronda Bessner

The recent development of scientific techniques which enable physicians to visualize the fetus, detect abnormalities and to treat the fetus *in utero*, has resulted in a radical transformation in the way pregnancy is perceived.[1] Medical technology such as ultrasound, amniocentesis and fetal heart monitors, as well as fetal surgery, have significantly altered the maternal/fetal relationship.[2] While many of the scientific techniques have been credited with "enhancing women's reproductive freedom," there is now an understanding that this new technology has been responsible for curtailing the autonomy of pregnant women.[3] In the past, both because of the inaccessible nature of the fetus as well as the paucity of knowledge of fetal development, the pregnant woman and the fetus were viewed as a single patient.[4] An examination of court decisions rendered in the past six or seven years reveals that the pregnant woman and her fetus are no longer considered as one entity but rather as two separate patients, with interests that may be in conflict or at cross-purposes.[5]

To date, the vehicles used by the state in Canada and the United States to curtail the acts of women during pregnancy have been child protection law, mental health legislation and criminal law. The state has sought to impose civil and criminal sanctions on women during their pregnancy, during the birthing process and subsequent to delivery.

It is the thesis of this paper that the responsibility of the woman to protect her fetus should be a moral and not a legal obligation. Imposing civil and criminal sanctions in such circumstances violates the rights of the woman to physical autonomy and self-determination and creates an adversarial relationship between the mother and her fetus and between the pregnant woman and her physician. In sum, imposing these legal sanctions serves as an impediment to the development of effective policies to protect the health of both the pregnant woman and her fetus.[6]

A DISCUSSION OF THE LAW

In Canada, Children's Aid Societies in several provinces have applied to the courts for an order that the fetus in question is a "child in need of protection" under the respective child welfare legislation. Child abuse laws which were never intended to apply to a woman's prenatal behaviour have been used by these agencies to justify their attempts to control the acts of pregnant women.[7] For example, in the 1987 case *Re Children's Aid Society of the City of Belleville*,[8] the C.A.S. sought such an order from the Ontario Provincial Court pursuant to the *Child and Family Services Act*.[9] The court stated that the following four factors indicated that "the unborn *child*" was "in need of protection":[10]

1. The pregnant woman, Linda T., had abdominal pain;

2. She had some discharge, which the court stated, "may or may not be normal in this particular situation";

3. She had spent a night in an underground parking lot; and

4. Linda T. had not sought obstetrical care.

Counsel for the pregnant woman argued that these problems were economically based. The court, however, refused to accept this explanation. Kirkland J. held that the fetus was a "child in need of protection" and was to be made a ward of the C.A.S. for three months,[11] which presumably was for the duration of the pregnancy. The court came to this conclusion despite the fact that the *Child and Family Services Act* defines "child" as a "*person* under the age of eighteen years."[12] In addition, the C.A.S. sought an order of committal under the Ontario *Mental Health Act*[13] to compel Linda T. to undergo "treatment" in the interests of the unborn child. Kirkland J. stated that the four factors enumerated above demonstrated that there was reasonable cause to believe that Linda T. suffered from a mental disorder of a nature and quality that would result in serious bodily harm to herself or another person.[14] The fetus, in the opinion of the court, constituted a person. As a result, Linda T. was detained until the birth of the child.

Conspicuously absent from the judgement in the *City of Belleville* was a discussion of the violation of the right of the woman to autonomy and bodily integrity. The court failed to acknowledge that the measures it imposed on Linda T. under the child welfare and mental health legislation constituted a fundamental violation of this woman's rights to privacy and to liberty to be protected from state control over her body.

A similar attempt to control a woman's conduct during gestation was in *Re A (in utero)*,[15] a 1990 decision of the Ontario Family Court. Without any notification to the pregnant woman, an application was made by the Children's Aid Society of Hamilton Wentworth under the *Child and Family Services Act* [16] for an interim order that the pregnant woman submit to prenatal care. The Crown also requested an order of wardship of the unborn "child," and an order requiring the pregnant woman to be detained in the hospital until the birth and to undergo all "necessary procedures" for the protection of the fetus. The C.A.S. argued that the husband was violent and had a criminal record; the couple had not adequately cared for their four other children; the woman was suffering from toxemia; the husband and wife had lied to the social workers about the prenatal care; and the social workers had been physically threatened by the husband for attempting to interfere with the pregnancy.[17]

The Ontario court refused to grant the relief sought by the C.A.S. Steinberg U.F.C.J. held that there was no provision in the *Child and Family Services Act* which accorded to "the fetus any status as a person" or a "right to protection."[18] The judge noted that had the parents been notified of the court proceedings, they likely would have fled the province.[19]

The court further stated that any attempt to protect the fetus necessarily involves a physical invasion of the pregnant woman. In the words of Judge Steinberg, it "is impossible in this case to take steps to protect the child without ultimately forcing the mother, under restraint if necessary, to undergo medical treatment and other processes, against her will."[20] Despite those statements prohibiting the state from intervening in the pregnancy, the court observed that this fetus had developed all the attributes of a person even though it was not a "person in law"; "the fetus can be likened to a person with a disability, perhaps deserving of protection."[21] According to Steinberg U.F.C.J.:[22]

> There is no doubt that the state has an interest in protecting those fetuses that mothers have decided to bring to full term, but the means and criteria for their protection had best be left to the legislature or Parliament and not to the discretion of the judiciary.

Thus, it was the court's view that if specific legislation authorizing intervention in pregnancy was enacted, the judiciary would be more willing to make orders that prescribed women's behaviour during gestation and childbirth.

This is precisely what some provinces have done. In New Brunswick, the *Family Services Act*[23] was amended to include an "unborn child" in the definition of "child." As a result, a New Brunswick court in a 1990 decision came to the determination that it was in the best interests of the fetus to impose a six month supervisory order on a pregnant woman.[24] Similarly, the Yukon Territory government included the following provision in the *Children's Act*[25] which authorized state intervention in pregnancy in the following circumstances:

> Where the Director has reasonable and probable grounds to believe and does believe that a fetus is being subjected to a serious risk or suffering from fetal alcohol syndrome or other congenital injury attributable to the pregnant woman subjecting herself during pregnancy to addictive or intoxicating substances, the Director may apply to a judge for an order requiring the woman to participate in such reasonable supervision or counselling as the order specifies in respect of her use of addictive or intoxicating substances. (emphasis added)

It was held in *Joe v. Yukon Territory Director of Family and Children's Services*[26] that this provision was unconstitutional on the grounds of vagueness — fetal alcohol syndrome was not defined in the legislation. The Yukon Territory Court stated that a citizen could not have her liberty rights infringed by legislation that was not specific.[27] Despite the fact that the Court held that the provision violated the right to liberty in Section 7 of the *Canadian Charter of Rights and Freedoms*,[28] it is implicit in the judgement that the court would have been predisposed to granting an order controlling the conduct of a pregnant woman had the terms in the legislation been precisely defined.

The British Columbia decision *Re Baby R*[29] is an example of the manner in which physicians and Children's Aid Societies seek to prescribe the behaviour of women during childbirth. A woman refused to follow her doctor's instructions to have her baby delivered by cesarean section. It was the doctor's opinion that a cesarean operation was necessary because of the likely complications of a vaginal birth; there was a "real danger of injury or death" if the child were delivered by natural childbirth.[30] As in the *City of Belleville*[31] case, the woman's doctor contacted the Family and Child Services Department who in turn initiated a lawsuit pursuant to the B.C. child welfare and mental health legislation. Without notification to the woman, the Superintendent of Family and Child Services instructed two police officers and two social workers to apprehend the unborn child and to ensure that the "emergency medical treatment" was performed.[32] Unaware of the actions of the Superintendent, the pregnant woman voluntarily consented to the cesarean section. However, immediately following the birth, the child was taken into custody of the state and placed in a foster home.[33]

The B.C. Supreme Court held that the Superintendent lacked the statutory authority to intervene in the pregnancy as the *Family and Child Services Act* defined "child" "as a person under nineteen years."[34] The court reasoned that as an age can not be acquired until after birth, the powers of the Superintendent are restricted to living children who have been delivered.[35] The court was critical of the fact that the baby was physically removed from the mother following the birth since the sole basis for the apprehension was the "presumed need"[36] for the cesarean birth. Despite these comments, the B.C. court, as in the cases discussed above, stated that in order to impinge upon a pregnant woman's rights, Parliament must enact legislation specifically addressed to this issue.[37]

In addition to the civil sanctions sought to be imposed on women through child welfare and mental health legislation, proponents of state intervention have recommended that criminal laws be enacted to punish women for inappropriate conduct during pregnancy. For instance, the Canada Law Reform Commission in a working paper entitled *Crimes Against the Fetus*[38] has proposed that the *Criminal Code*[39] be amended to include the following provision:

> *1) Everyone commits a crime who...*
>> *b) being a pregnant woman, purposely causes destruction or serious harm to her fetus by any act or by failing to make reasonable provision for assistance in respect of her delivery.*

This proposal has been the subject of serious criticism and organizations such as the Canadian Bar Association have recommended a complete ban on judicial intervention during gestation and childbirth.[40]

A review of the decisions rendered in Canada demonstrates that the state, through child welfare legislation and mental health legislation, has attempted to intervene in pregnancies. Moreover, there have been proposals that the *Criminal Code* be amended to ensure that women be subject to criminal convictions for conduct during their pregnancy that adversely affects their fetuses.

An examination of the legislation and the court decisions in the United States reveals that state intervention in pregnancy has been extensive. By order of civil courts, women have been compelled to undergo cesarean sections, forced to submit to blood transfusions and detained in hospitals.[41] In addition, state legislatures such as Minnesota[42] and Oklahoma[43] have enacted laws that require physicians to report women who use drugs during pregnancy. Failure to report constitutes a misdemeanour. Furthermore, women have been criminally convicted for behaviour during pregnancy.[44] Women have been arrested in Massachusetts, Connecticut, Ohio, Illinois, Indiana, and Michigan.[45]

POLICY ARGUMENTS AGAINST JUDICIAL INTERVENTION IN PREGNANCIES

State intervention in pregnancy constitutes a serious violation of a woman's right to bodily integrity and self-determination. Compelling a woman to undergo a cesarean section or fetal surgery, ordering a pregnant woman to submit to a blood transfusion, and detaining a woman to ensure that she complies with her obstetrician's instructions constitutes a deprivation of a woman's fundamental rights. Many proponents of state intervention appear reluctant to openly acknowledge that access to the fetus involves an infringement of the woman's physical autonomy.[46]

The right of a competent adult to refuse medical treatment, an important principle of tort law, is premised on respect for an individual's autonomy and bodily integrity.[47] A physician who treats a patient without his or her informed consent is subject to an action in battery.[48] Court decisions which impose sanctions on a woman for refusing to comply with an obstetrician's instructions constitutes a fundamental violation of a woman's right to decide whether or not to receive treatment.[49] As Annas asks rhetorically in *Forced Cesareans: The Most Unkindest Cut of All*,[50] "do we really want to restrain, forcibly medicate and operate on a competent refusing adult?" Tolton argues that:[51]

> *Even though the conceptus is greatly affected by the woman's decision, society must accept the fact that its relationship with the conceptus must be mediated by the woman within whose body it is. Given the physical reality of the situation, the decision maker must be the pregnant woman, not doctors, social workers, or even judges.*

Judges who compel pregnant women to submit to treatment against their will are imposing burdens and medical risks on women that are not placed on other members of society.[52] For example, a cesarean operation constitutes major abdominal surgery — the risk of maternal mortality from a cesarean is four times higher than that of a vaginal delivery.[53]

It is undeniable that virtually all acts of the pregnant woman have an effect on the fetus as the fetus is physically dependent on the woman for its development and survival.[54] Given this fact, legislators could impose liability on women for any behaviour that could potentially have a detrimental effect on the fetus, such as engaging in sexual intercourse, failing to eat properly, smoking, using prescription or non-prescription drugs, drinking coffee, drinking alcohol, exposure to workplace hazards or infectious diseases, or using a general anaesthetic to induce labour.[55] These restrictions on the conduct of pregnant women could conceivably be extended by the state to all fertile women of childbearing age as, for example, it is argued that alcohol consumption can have an adverse effect on the fetus before the woman is even aware that she is pregnant.[56] Thus, the list of activities that may be proscribed affects everything a woman does — what she eats, how she earns her livelihood, how and whether she moves, and her sexual behaviour.[57] As stated by a commentator, if the current trend persists, pregnant women "will live in constant fear that any accident or 'error' in judgement, could become the basis of a civil suit or criminal prosecution.[58] Moreover, given new developments in fetal therapy and surgery, state intervention in pregnancy is susceptible to even more dangerous expansion."[59]

It is essential to understand that many women are denied procedural due process in circumstances in which the state intervenes in pregnancy. For instance, in the 1990 case *Re A*[60] discussed above, the woman had no knowledge that the Children's Aid Society had made an application to the court to compel her to submit to prescribed prenatal care. In the event of noncompliance, the C.A.S. requested that the pregnant woman be detained in the hospital until the birth and be forced to submit to all "necessary procedures" for the protection of the fetus. Because she was not notified of the court proceedings, the woman was not present at the hearing nor did she have counsel to represent her interests. It is also important to note that because of the emergency nature of many hearings, a judge is often compelled to decide in an unduly short period of time whether to order surgery for a competent unconsenting adult.[61] As Rhoden states, judges are not "likely to hear lucid constitutional arguments from one in the hospital, in the sweating agonies of labor, or from her counsel appointed one hour before the hearing."[62]

One must ask the proponents of state intervention, who is the appropriate individual or body to make medical decisions on behalf of the pregnant woman. U.S. cases demonstrate that the refusal of a pregnant woman to follow her doctor's instructions is, in some circumstances, the wisest course of action.[63] Doctors are not infallible and physician prediction of fetal harm is not always accurate.[64] It is essential that the pregnant woman, rather than the physician, make the ultimate decision regarding appropriate medical treatment as it is the woman, not the physician, who will bear the burden of an erroneous diagnosis and prognosis.[65] Furthermore, a strong argument can be made that it is the pregnant woman who is best situated to make this complex assessment and to evaluate the competing pressures with which she is confronted.[66] The decisions of a woman during her pregnancy are dependent upon her "individual values," her "life circumstances," and "uncertain probabilities of daily risk."[67] The vast majority of women care profoundly about the well-being of the child they will bear and will avoid any harm to their fetus.[68]

It must also be acknowledged that the family entity is adversely affected in circumstances in which the state imposes such legal responsibilities upon the pregnant woman.[69] A review of both legislation and judicial decisions in the last decades demonstrates a reluctance on the part of the state to intervene in the ongoing decisions of the family. Historically, there has been an assumption that the family will make decisions that are in its best interests.[70] As an author observes, the state's "willingness to target the pregnant drug-user or to permit doctors to perform cesarean sections over a pregnant woman's objections seems inconsistent with this reluctance to invade the privacy of the family."[71]

In terms of the Courts' analysis in the decisions that have been rendered, the conceptualization of the problem as a conflict between maternal and fetal interests is counterproductive as it undermines the importance of the connection between the mother and her fetus.[72] As is stated by Johnsen: [73]

> *Allowing the state to control women's actions in the name of fetal rights reflects a view of the fetus as an entity separate from the woman, with interests that are hostile to her interests. In fact, by granting rights to the fetus assertible against the pregnant woman, and thus depriving the woman of decision-making autonomy, the state affirmatively acts to create an adversarial relationship between the woman and the fetus.*

Similarly, in a *Harvard Law Review* article, the author contends that by "characterizing the issue of fetal endangerment as a choice between women's autonomy and fetal health, the rights framework has led to policies that effectively protect neither."[74]

State intervention in pregnancy is also responsible for creating an adversarial relationship between the woman and her obstetrician.[75] A woman might decide to withhold important medical information from her physician or refuse to seek prenatal care if she thinks her doctor will report her to state authorities.[76] This may occur if the pregnant woman believes her doctor will have a lawsuit initiated against her for not following the prescribed medical advice, for example, to adhere to dietary, exercise and travel restrictions, to refrain from engaging in sexual intercourse, or to submit to a cesarean or other surgical procedure.

As the U.S. experience demonstrates, criminal prosecutions and civil actions "have the effect of deterring women from using the very health related services that will most benefit themselves and their children."[77] Women who believe that their decision-making autonomy and physical integrity will not be respected may choose not to deliver their babies in hospitals and not to seek prenatal care. Health problems of the fetus may as a result not be detected which obviously runs counter to the objectives of those who advocate state intervention in pregnancy.[78]

It has been asserted that women's rights to equality are violated in circumstances in which the state imposes sanctions on women for their conduct during pregnancy.[79] One must ask why the interests of pregnant women are treated differently from analogous interests of other individuals in society? There is no obligation in law to be a good samaritan. Is it equitable to impose more onerous obligations on a pregnant woman than society is willing to impose on parents in general?[80] No similar duty of physical subordination is owed by parents to their existing children.[81] As an American writer argues:[82]

> ...Some courts have required that the pregnant woman have a cesarean operation — a procedure that is risky and physically invasive. Yet, we have not been willing to require of parents that they be required to donate kidneys to children who might otherwise die in the absence of a kidney transplant.

Laws in both Canada and the United States do not oblige parents to undergo surgical procedures and other medical treatment to benefit their born children. As maintained by Goldberg, to compel a pregnant woman to submit to medical treatment against her will to benefit the fetus not only endows the fetus with greater rights than the woman but also gives the fetus more rights than are currently accorded to existing children.[83]

Nor are similar legal obligations imposed on prospective fathers. Analogous behaviour engaged in by men which adversely affects the fetus is not subject to civil or criminal liability. For instance, studies indicate that ingesting substances such as alcohol, morphine or methadone may damage the sperm.[84] Moreover, a fetus may be affected if subjected to heavy smoking of his/her prospective father.[85] King reports that in a California case, the mother, not the father, was criminally prosecuted, in part, for engaging in sexual intercourse during the pregnancy. As King observes, "the last time I examined the issue, the act of intercourse required two people."[86]

CONCLUSION

As is argued in this paper, a pregnant woman's responsibility to care for her fetus should be a moral and not a legal obligation. State intervention in pregnancy constitutes a deprivation of a woman's right to bodily integrity and self-determination. Moreover, measures imposed by the state create an adversarial relationship between the woman and her fetus, and between the woman and her physician. Some fetuses may be born with defects and some fetuses may even die. However, the measures currently imposed on pregnant women in North America through child abuse statutes, mental health legislation and the criminal law undermine the development of effective policies such as education for the protection of both the pregnant woman and her fetus.

NOTES

1　N.K. Rhoden, "The judge in the delivery room: The emergence of court-ordered cesareans" 1986, 74 *Calif. L. Rev.* 1951.

2　S. Goldberg, "Medical choices during pregnancy: Whose decision is it anyway" 1989, 41 *Rutgers L. Rev.* 591.

3　D. Johnsen, "The creation of fetal rights: conflicts with women's constitutional rights to liberty, privacy, and equal protection" 1986 *Yale L.J.* 599 at 609.

4　P. King, "Should mom be constrained in the best interests of the fetus" 1989, 13 *Nova Law Review* 393 at 396.

5　*Supra.*, note 3, at 599-600, and *Supra.*, note 2, at 591-592.

6　See "Rethinking motherhood: Feminist theory and state regulation of pregnancy" 1990, *Harv. L. Rev.* 1325 at 1326, 1333, 1337.

7　See K. Moss, "Substance abuse during pregnancy" 1990, 13 *Harvard Women's Law Journal* 278 at 285-286.

8　1987, 59 O.R. (2d) 204 (Ont. Prov. Ct.)

9　1984, c. 55, s. 37.

10　*Supra*, note 8, at 205-206.

11 *Ibid.*, at 206.
12 *Supra*, note 9.
13 R.S.O. 1980, c. 262, s. 10.
14 *Supra*, note 8, at 207-208.
15 (1990), 75 O.R. (2d) 82.
16 *Supra*, note 9.
17 *Supra*, note 15, at 84-87.
18 *Ibid.*, at 88-89.
19 *Ibid.*, at 87.
20 *Ibid.*, at 92.
21 *Ibid.*, at 90.
22 *Ibid.*, at 92.
23 S.N.B. 1986, c. F-2.2.
24 *The Minister of Health and Community Service v. A.D.* (1990), 109 N.B.R. (2d) 192 (Q.B.).
25 S.Y.T. 1984, c.2, s.134 (1).
26 (1986), 5 B.C.L.R. (2d) 267 (Yuk. Terr. Sup. Ct.)
27 *Ibid.*
28 Section 7 of the *Charter* provides: Everyone has the right to life, liberty and security of the person and
    the right not to be deprived thereof except in accordance with the principles of fundamental justice.28.
29 (1988) 15 R.F.L. (3d) 225 (B.C.S.C.).
30 *Ibid.*, at 229.
31 *Supra*, note 8.
32 *Supra*, note 29, at 230.
33 *Ibid.*
34. *Ibid.*, at 234.
35 *Ibid.*, at 237.
36 Ibid., at 234.
37 Ibid., at 237.
38 Working Paper 58, 1989 at 51.
39 R.S.C. 1985, c. C-46.
40 *Judicial Intervention During Gestation and Childbirth,* Background Paper, November 1990.
41 Supra, note 4, at 608. See, for example, *Re A,* A.2d 611 (D.C. App. 1987) vacated and reh'g
    granted 539 A.2d 203 (1988) (en banc); *Jefferson v. Griffin Spalding County Hospital,* 247 Ga. 86,
    274 S.E. 2d 457 (1981) and *Raleigh Fitkin-Paul Morgan Memorial Hospital v. Anderson,* 42 N.J.
    421, 201 A.2d 537, Cert. denied, 377 U.S. 985 (1964).
42 Minn. Stat. 626.556 (1988).
43 Okla. Stat. Ann. tit.21, 846 (West 1989).
44 Supra, note 7, at 280.
45 *Ibid.*, at 285.
46 *Supra*, note 2, at 592.
47 *Supra*, note 2, at 617.
48 A. Linden, *Canadian Tort Law* (Toronto: Butterworths Co., 1977) at 59; and *Supra*, note 1, at 1969.

49 *Supra*, note 2, at 594.
50 (1982) Hastings Center Report 16 at 18.
51 C. Tolton, "Medicolegal implications of constitutional states for the unborn: 'Ambulatory chalices' or 'priorities and aspirations'" (1988), 47 *U. of Tor. Fac. Law Rev.* 1 at 38.
52 *Supra*, note 1, at 2029.
53 *Ibid.*, at 1958.
54 *Supra*, note 3, at 605-606; and *Supra.*, note 6, at 1340.
55 *Supra*, note 3, 606-607.
56 *Supra*, note 7 at 288-289.
57 *Supra*, note 4 at 397.
58 *Supra*, note 3 at 607.
59 *Ibid.*, at 608-609.
60 *Supra*, note 15.
61 *Supra*, note 1, at 1952.
62 *Ibid.*, at 2029.
63 *Supra*, note 2, at 604.
64 *Ibid.*, at 604 and 623; *Supra*, note 50, at 17; and *Supra*, note 4, at 402.
65 *Supra*, note 4, at 402.
66 *Ibid.;* and *Supra.*, note 3, at 613.
67 *Supra*, note 3, at 613.
68 *Ibid.*
69 *Supra*, note 4, at 403.
70 *Ibid.*
71 *Supra*, note 6, at 1337.
72 *Ibid.*, at 1336.
73 *Supra*, note 3, at 613.
74 *Supra*, note 6, at 1337.
75 *Supra*, note 50, at 18.
76 *Supra*, note 2, at 622-623.
77 *Supra*, note 7, at 288.
78 *Supra*, note 2, at 620.
79 *Supra*, note 4, at 399.
80 *Ibid.*, at 400-401.
81 *Supra*, note 2, at 594-595.
82 *Supra*, note 4, at 400. and 398 See also *Supra*, note 50, at 17..
83 *Supra*, note 2, at 621.
84 *Supra*, note 7, at 286.
85 *Supra*, note 4, at 400.
86 *Ibid.*

30

SOME REFLECTIONS ON "SURROGACY"

Susan Sherwin

First, I want to spend a moment on terminology. "Surrogacy" is the term most often used to describe the arrangements by which a woman (commonly called the "surrogate mother") agrees to become pregnant, carry the embryo to term, and, after giving birth, surrender custody of the child to the contracting father or couple.[1] The term "surrogate mother" is a misnomer; the woman who is assigned this position is the birth mother, and she is, therefore, the biological mother of the child in question, having (usually) both conceived and gestated it in her body. The only sort of surrogate or "stand-in" role she occupies is that of surrogate wife to the man who contracts her reproductive "services" and supplies the sperm for fertilization. Even when the egg that is fertilized is obtained from another woman (who may be either a third party donor or the woman who plans to become the adoptive mother of the resulting child), the so-called surrogate still has a significant biological mothering role to play. In such complicated circumstances, where the birth mother, genetic mother, and social mother roles may all be distinct, it is a difficult and open question to determine which contribution makes someone a "real" rather than "surrogate" mother.

While this fussing about terminology may seem to be "mere" semantic quibbling on the part of a philosopher, I think it is important, since the terms we use are revealing of the assumptions that govern our thought on this practice. To describe the woman who conceives, carries and gives birth to the developing embryo as a "surrogate" is to begin with the assumption that her reproductive role is marginal and mechanical, that of a place holder rather than a central participant. It declares from the start that she is not the "real" mother, but only a surrogate, and, therefore, it conveys the message that women's biological contributions to the development of babies are somehow interchangeable and peripheral. I object to such assumptions, and hence, I recommend adopting a different terminology. I will speak instead of "contractual pregnancy"; this terminology makes explicit the relationships at work and the centrality of women's reproductive role to these arrangements.

How, then, are we to approach the revised question of whether and how to "regulate contractual pregnancies"? As an ethicist, it seems to me that the first task is to determine what is morally relevant in this matter, i.e., what are the ethical considerations we should bring to bear? In my book, *No Longer Patient: Feminist Ethics and Health Care*,[2] I argue that when we are trying to determine the ethical acceptability of a practice, we must attend to its role within the existing patterns of *oppression* in our society. Following Iris Young,[3] I understand oppression to be a form of injustice that is characterized by any combination of exploitation, marginalization, powerlessness, cultural imperialism and violence that are directed at an identifiable social group. Oppression is a socially based constraint which does not always require malevolent intention to be effective; the term also "refers to the vast and deep injustices some groups suffer as a consequence of often unconscious assumptions and reactions of well-meaning people in ordinary interactions, media and cultural stereotypes, and structural features of bureaucratic hierarchies and market mechanisms — in short, the normal processes of everyday life.... oppressions are systematically reproduced in major economic, political, and cultural institutions."[4]

I begin my analysis, then, with the feminist assumption that there exist systemic forms of oppression in our society, by which matters of gender, as well as race, class, sexual orientation, ethnicity, age, ability status and other such features, affect an individual's opportunities and position in society. As well, my discussion is informed by the corresponding feminist belief that oppression is morally objectionable and, therefore, it should be reduced and, ultimately, eliminated.

Thus, in my view, when we set out to evaluate the ethical acceptability of a practice, or when we try to determine the best policy regarding a certain social practice, we must attend to the question of how this practice contributes to existing forms of oppression in society: does it (a) help to undermine and reduce oppressive forces, (b) reinforce and support them, or (c) is it neutral with respect to current patterns of oppression? The question here, then, is how, in particular, would institutionalizing contractual pregnancy via some form of regulation contribute to existing forms of oppression in our society? Any attempt to regulate contractual pregnancy that permits some such arrangements will amount to a degree of social endorsement and tolerance and will lend the practice credibility and legitimacy. Hence, we need to decide whether prohibition or some other form of regulation will be most effective at reducing existing oppressions relative to the effects achieved by alternative policies.

In order to determine what the effects of a regulatory policy in this area might be, it is important to understand the social context in which the policy will operate. A state-authorized, regulated practice of contractual pregnancy is most likely to affect the existing forms of oppression that are based on gender and class; thus, I shall concentrate on these two forms of oppression. It is important to note, though, that the influence of such a policy may also be felt in the areas of oppression based on matters of race and ethnicity, disability and sexual orientation and we might well expect it to have repercussions in widespread social attitudes towards children. With respect to gender, the potential effects of a socially accepted practice of contractual pregnancy are compounded by the fact that this is but one practice among many which are designed to eliminate or circumvent a woman's infertility. It is part of a massive medical, legal and social effort to ensure that every woman have the opportunity to "mother" no matter what physical impediments may be present. It is a reflection of the assumption that raising children is of central importance to women and is a primary element of heterosexual marriage. Along with other new reproductive practices, contractual pregnancy is evolving in the face of enormous media and political interest which anticipates, endorses and stresses the urgency couples feel about their desire to reproduce by whatever means are available; such attention conveys without question a strong social message about the centrality of reproduction in the lives of women and couples.

Moreover, it is a practice based on the assumption that it is very important that if men choose, they have the opportunity to father genetically related children. So, if their wives cannot provide them, then some other woman, some "surrogate," can be counted on to accomplish this end. It is a practice that helps to perpetuate the view that fatherhood is chiefly determined by a man's genetic contribution,[5] while motherhood is a matter of fulfilling the socially prescribed role of nurturer and caregiver. The asymmetry that is presumed in the reproductive contributions required of men and women in order to qualify as parents in these circumstances is quite clear. It is an asymmetry rooted in the traditionally unjust sexual division of labour that still underlies men's privilege and women's subordination in society. The implicit devaluing of the contribution of the biological mother, in which her role is commodified within the terms of a commercial transaction, resonates with historical devaluing of women's reproductive roles that dates back at least to Aristotle's "flower pot" theory of pregnancy.[6]

It is important to recognize that most contractual pregnancies are ultimately about relationships among women. The usual pattern is that one woman agrees to become pregnant and, after childbirth, to give up her parental rights to another woman who will then become the child's adoptive mother; hence, the arrangements governing this practice should concentrate on clarifying these women's relationships to one another and to the child. But, in the reality of contractual arrangements, these relationships are commonly determined and mediated by men, specifically by the man who is the biological father and the husband of the adopting mother. He is the one who retains parental status no matter what custody decision is finally made by the birth mother and, in the event that she does have second thoughts about surrendering her maternal rights, it is he, not his wife, who will have standing in any courtroom deciding custody. These are the background conditions in which contractual pregnancy arrangements are negotiated and carried out. Within the current social environment, it is simply not possible to assure gender equality of all participants, which would be a requirement for any acceptable practice of contractual pregnancy. More seriously, it is by no means clear that contractual pregnancy arrangements will help to advance our social expectations to a point where gender equality in reproduction would be the case in such arrangements (though at least one feminist, Carmen Shavel, argues that it would in her book *Birth Power*)[7]. It seems more likely that contractual pregnancy arrangements will deepen and further entrench the gender inequality inherent in current attitudes towards reproduction; that is, they are more likely to deepen the existing oppression of women than to reduce it.

In matters of class, it has often been observed that contractual pregnancy arrangements almost always involve couples whose economic status is middle class or above who contract with a woman whose background is working class or below to produce a child for them. There is an inherent inequality in these respective positions that cannot be easily overcome. The vulnerability of poor women to exploitation by those who are more advantaged cannot be denied or ignored. Women with few marketable skills, or even skilled women at a time of deep recession, may find that their reproductive or sexual services are the only thing they have available to sell. In a hostile economy, many women find themselves with all too few economic choices, and they may well be forced by circumstances to agree to become impregnated in order to receive the financial compensation that is customary in these arrangements. Parallel arguments could, however, be applied to many other sources of income for women: e.g., it seems probable that the only way we find women willing to clean other people's homes, interrupt strangers' dinners with unwelcome telemarketing calls, or serve in a fast food chain is because they need the money that such employment will bring them. Clearly, there are many ways besides contractual pregnancy in which women are exploited in our economy. While some theorists may want to object to all forms of demeaning or mind-numbing employment as exploitative, I shall not here try to take on all of capitalism, but will instead explain why contractual pregnancy poses a particular worry that distinguishes it from other forms of economic exploitation.

What makes contractual pregnancy especially suspect is that it involves a different form of labour than is covered by our usual employment relationships. For one thing, it involves significant physical and psychological demands, for pregnancy involves dramatic physiological, hormonal and social changes in a woman's life. Full term pregnancies engage a woman in perhaps the most intimate of all human relationships as she carries a fetus past the stages of quickening and viability to the point where it becomes a recognizably other being who is in constant contact and interaction with her. Experience has shown that not all women are able to simply sever the emotional bonds generated by this twenty-four hour a day intimacy, and "give over" the baby after birth to be raised by others. If we wanted to protect women from the inherent risks of this practice, it is difficult to see how we might do so within the resources provided by legal conventions. Because there are no other models for this relationship and the effects it produces on the mother and fetus, the relationship cannot be simply reduced to others that have been successfully covered by legal contracts.

With other exploitative jobs, women have the opportunity to quit if they find the working conditions intolerable; the availability of unemployment insurance, and the prospects of other work can make resignation a realistic protection against excessive exploitation for most other "jobs." With contractual pregnancy, it is not so easy to resign. Once pregnant, and especially once the fetus reaches the stage of quickening where its distinct existence becomes a felt reality for a woman, it is usually not possible to end the pregnancy (and it is especially not possible if the reason for her second thoughts is that she has become emotionally attached to the developing fetus). Nor, however, is she likely to be in a position to keep the child upon birth if her initial reason for agreeing to the contract was financial need. An additional child will add significantly to her already high financial burden, so, even if contracts are written in such a way as to allow women to change their minds for some period after birth, if women who participate are the ones who most need the money (as is usually the case), they may find themselves unable to provide for a new child; hence, they may have no real option but to comply with the terms of the contract despite their current reluctance. Existing oppression of poor women makes them vulnerable to economic exploitation and contractual pregnancy arrangements take advantage of their oppressed status by further exploiting them. Rather than reducing the vulnerability of poor women to such exploitative arrangements, legitimizing contractual pregnancies in which women are offered a token "fee" for their services takes advantage of their economic disadvantage and helps to maintain the economic disparity from which they begin.

Perhaps, then, the ideal would be to allow such arrangements but avoid the monetary dimension. Refuse to allow contractual mothers to receive any payment for their "inconvenience" and so rely only on women who are willing to participate for reasons of altruism or curiosity (as several authors have proposed when the fear of economic exploitation is raised). This, too, is problematic, for women may still be coerced by circumstances into participation: part of the socialization of women is to be altruistic, to be self-sacrificing and "caring." It is all too easy for contractual pregnancy arrangements to draw on this character trait that is part of women's socialization for their subordinate social position and persuade individuals to make this very generous move for no profit whatsoever. This hardly seems to be an improvement. Moreover, the fear that women's socialization towards subordinate roles is at issue here can also call into question the consent of the other woman involved, i.e., the wife of the man whose sperm are used to father the child. If her husband is eager to have a child of his own genetic heritage, and she is unable to bear such a child, a wife who feels her marriage depends on her cooperation may also feel little freedom to resist these arrangements.

Nonetheless, despite these overwhelming odds against the likelihood of anyone developing a non-exploitative, non-oppressive contractual pregnancy arrangement, it is at least possible that some specific contractual pregnancy arrangement, looked at in isolation, may seem to be reasonable and defensible. It may be that the contracting couple is well meaning and well informed in their desire to reproduce. There may be no reason to fault their sincerity or to challenge their motivation, and it is certainly not their fault that there is economic need in the world and that they are in a position to relieve some of that need by contracting for a service they badly want. There may even be good evidence to expect them to become loving and effective parents if all goes according to plan. Further, it may well be the case that the contracting birth mother is also well informed and willing. She would resent the description of her as exploited and consider this to be a patronizing distortion of her motivation, which may entail elements of altruism, personal satisfaction, and a realistic choice of her income options and personal needs. In other words, specific contractual pregnancy arrangements can appear to be positive experiences for all parties directly concerned — everybody benefits: the social parents, the biological mother and the child produced. I do not mean to deny the possibility of this outcome, though I believe that the evidence to date suggests it is, at best, very rare.

My point is that social practices are sometimes more than the sum of their parts — the effects of a practice or policy may extend beyond the well being of the contracting parties. When trying to determine an appropriate social policy about regulating contractual pregnancies, we need to take into account not only the interests of the direct participants, but also the interests of society at large and consider how this policy fits into a larger social system where all women are oppressed and vulnerable, and where women who are poor, belong to racial minorities, have disabilities, identify themselves as lesbian, and so on are especially oppressed. Within such a culture, a general practice of contractual pregnancy seems more likely to support and reinforce deeply sexist, racist, classist and heterosexualist attitudes than to undermine them.

Women are reduced to purely biological roles on the one hand, and to caregivers on the other, as the true meaning of motherhood is debated, while fatherhood seems to be clearly defined and constant if largely a matter of genetic input and sufficient wealth to negotiate suitable arrangements. Implicitly, there is a commitment to the importance of genetic relation on the part of men and the insignificance of this factor on the part of women. Custom-made children are created at significant expense while existing, "hard to place" children remain homeless. And heterosexual, two-person marriages are to be completed by the addition of special order children, reinforcing the norms of what constitutes a "family" while other sorts of living arrangements (e.g., same sex couples, single parents, and other sorts of "differently constructed" families) continue to be treated as anomalous and undeserving of any sort of special arrangement.

The final difficulty I would like to raise is the degree of autonomy expressed by the women who become involved in these sorts of contractual arrangements. The premise of any contract is that each party is rational and autonomous and their signature is evidence that they believe the contract will best serve their interests. I accept that participation in these arrangements can be a rational and desirable choice on the part of each participant. What I object to are the conditions under which the choice is made and the narrow options available to some of the participants in this scheme. So long as women must make their reproductive decisions under conditions of inequality and limited autonomy, it is a mistake to look only at the particular moment of reproductive decision-making and call it rational or autonomous. Affluent men set the terms of participation for both their wives and the contracting birth mothers in this non-conventional reproductive arrangement; the cooperation of the women involved cannot be separated from the matter of their relative economic and social disadvantage. Contractual pregnancies pose significant ethical problems that cannot be addressed simply by treating them like any other contractual arrangement, by providing the authority of the state and its courts to ensure contracts are fairly prepared and enforced. Contracts are legal instruments designed to govern exchanges between two roughly equally situated parties, but in the face of existing gender, class and race oppressions, the parties are not equally situated. Moreover, contractual pregnancy arrangements, if legalized and accepted, are more likely to exacerbate such inequalities than to reduce them. Thus, at least in the current social and historical moment, feminists should resist any form of regulation of contractual pregnancies other than prohibition.

NOTES

1 This paper was presented to a conference on Law and Contemporary Affairs sponsored by the Faculty of Law, University of Toronto, Feb. 5, 1993, as part of a panel on "Regulating Surrogacy."

2 Susan Sherwin, *No Longer Patient: Feminist Ethics and Health Care* Philadelphia: Temple University Press, 1992.

3 Iris Marion Young, *Justice and the Politics of Difference* Princeton: Princeton University Press, 1990.

4 Ibid., 41.

5   That is, if he chooses to claim this genetic connection. It is important to note that fatherhood is a matter of both genetic contribution and claimed relation; men who father children outside of marriage, and those who provide sperm for use in anonymous artificial insemination arrangements may not be socially construed as the fathers of their offspring. I owe my recognition of this complexity to Margrit Eichler.

6   In the "flower pot theory," women are assigned the same passive role and contribution to reproduction as a flower pot; i.e., the important and distinctive contribution belongs to the man who plants his seed in her, and she merely provides the space and necessary nutrients for growth. For a description of Aristotle's "flower-pot" theory, see Caroline Whitbeck, "Theories of Sex Difference." *Philosophical Forum* 5(1, 2): 54-80.

7   Carmen Shavel, *Birth Power: The Case for Surrogacy* New Haven: Yale University Press, 1989.

31

REFLECTIONS ON THE "TEMPORARY USE OF NORMALLY FUNCTIONING UTERI"

Margrit Eichler

In his 1988 address[1] to the Annual Meeting of the Pacific Coast Obstetrical and Gynecological Society, the president shared his thoughts on reproductive surrogacy with his audience.[2] While on the one hand he offered his sympathy to "barren women" who are condemned to remain childless, he put forward as the solution to this problem disembodied "uteri" who will produce, in a number of ways, children for these women. These "normally functioning uteri," of "'off-duty' gestational specialists" could help "women who seek the bliss of motherhood." The uteri would provide a "safe uterine haven" for, among others, the fetuses of women who have additional risks to "the risk of death or disability innate to pregnancy itself." Such risk is of no concern when it applies to these uteri. Quite to the contrary, "Reproductive surrogacy... has the immediate capacity to accomplish more for mankind [sic] in these areas than essentially any currently available technique."

The speech exemplifies the degree to which we have already come to accept preconception arrangements. Yet we know little about the people who are involved in these services, and next to nothing about Canadians involved in these arrangements. This is as true for the "uteri" as it is for the "barren women" — who are most usually wives to *men* who engage in these arrangements. There is much speculation and discussion but little concrete evidence. Various computer searches on the issue turned up well over 100 references.[3] Of these, two contained some solid information about people who participate in such arrangements. The others were mostly legal, philosophical, ethical, theological or journalistic reflections of the issue in general, or with one or two specific cases.[4] While some of these contributions are thoughtful and important in their own right, empirical evidence is sorely needed. Because there is no literature that provides comparative information on Canadian cases, every shred of data is of some use. This paper contains some such shreds.

THE HIDDEN NATURE OF THE PHENOMENON

In 1988, the Law Reform Commission of Canada asked me to conduct a small study on the incidence of preconception arrangements involving Canadians.[5] Our main question was a simple one: do Canadians participate in preconception arrangements for the production of children? The simple answer to this question is yes, they do, but it is exceedingly difficult to determine to what degree or in what manner.

To come up with even this answer was not easy. First we talked with lawyers (lawyers may be involved in drawing up the agreements). One of the lawyers suggested that we poll all family court judges, because they are involved in the adoption process. Taking this advice, we did poll all Ontario family court judges. A 75 percent response rate to our questionnaire resulted in identifying only 2 cases for us. One of the judges commented:

> *If you have the consent of the natural mother and the natural father and the adopting parents both agreeing, both sign the application... everything is dandy. What is wrong with it? You do not even bother to go any deeper than that. Everyone has signed and everyone agrees and away it goes.*

Unsatisfied, we engaged in an exhaustive search of popular media, talked with social workers across the country, who, with one other source, were most knowledgeable and helpful. We also contacted every child and family service in every province and territory and talked with other government officials, adoption agencies and services across the country, academics who had published on the issue (or were currently researching it), medical personnel, various other associations, centers, legal bodies, marriage and mediation counsellors, key informants who fell outside any of the categories so far listed. Finally, we attended a conference in which several sessions dealt with the issue. All of these efforts resulted in very skimpy information — we identified 42 cases through these sources.

There was one source that provided some substantial information: American agencies specializing in the arrangement of preconception agreements. We identified a minimum of 76 cases involving Canadians from 11[6] different American agencies. In all instances, we can assume that we are underestimating the actual incidence, but we do not know by what factor. The major American agency, Noel Keane's, with two centers (the Infertility Center in New York, and that in Dearborne, Michigan) allowed us access to their files.[7] The data in the next section are all drawn from these files.

Overall, we identified 118 cases involving Canadians.[8] These figures include commercial as well as non-commercial, privately arranged preconception arrangements for the production of children. Although this is a small number, this includes cases only until 1988, when the Law Reform Commission project was carried out. Presumably, there have been new ones since then.

Further, cases do not equal people. Cases were counted if any of the main actors — commissioned woman or commissioning man or couple — were Canadians. If it was the commissioned woman, she was most likely to be married, probably still had parents alive who would be grandparents of the child and highly likely to have had one or more children before engaging in an agreement — she had to be, after all, a "gestational specialist of proved ability."[9] If it was the commissioning man or couple, they might have parents still alive who would be grandparents of the child. The commissioning couple might have other children in the family.[10] If the entire case was arranged in Canada, these numbers would multiply. Therefore, each case in which a child was actually born is likely to involve up to three sets of grandparents, various siblings, spouses, cousins, aunts, uncles, nephews, nieces, as well as professionals involved in the arrangement.

A PARTIAL UNVEILING: DATA ON CANADIANS INVOLVED IN PRECONCEPTION AGREEMENTS AT KEANE'S AGENCY

Mr. Keane's willingness to share the information in his files provided a unique opportunity to obtain some systematic information about one group of

Canadians involved in preconception agreements. Since there are no commercial surrogacy brokers in Canada comparable to the American agencies, and there are a number of such agencies in the Unites States, trying to obtain a child by becoming a client of an American agency has become a new form of cross-border shopping for Canadians. Our telephone survey of American surrogacy agencies uncovered 76 cases involving Canadians as of 1988. The number of babies born in the U.S. via preconception arrangements[11] until that time has been put at "nearly six hundred" (U.S., 1988: 267). This suggests that about 13 percent of all cases at U.S. surrogacy agencies involved Canadian clients. A 1992 report puts the current U.S. figure at 4,000 (Charo, 1992).

The information we obtained is, of course, only as good as that in the files. Since all data were collected anonymously, we could neither fill the gaps when information was missing nor check its accuracy. Overall, we have comparable information on 32 cases. All of these involve Canadians as social parents.[12]

A NOTE ON TERMINOLOGY

Most feminists do not use the term surrogate mother, because — as has been observed again and again — these women are real mothers, even though they are planning to give up their child at birth. Sherwin (this volume) uses the term "contractual pregnancy" to describe the process. I have elsewhere used the term "preconception contracts for the production of children."[13] In our report to the Law Reform Commission, we identified the commissioned woman as the "contractual mother" and the commissioning man as the "father." Upon reflection, I have come to the conclusion that these terms are inappropriate, and have hence changed my terminology here. Not all of the women who are commissioned for a pregnancy actually give birth, and not all of the men who commission a child actually obtain one. To use parental terms, then, is inappropriate in both instances. It focuses our attention on those agreements·in which there is a "successful" outcome — that is, a child is actually born. One of the most surprising things we realized when looking at the data is the existence of people involved in these arrangements who may never become parents, but whose lives will nevertheless have been intimately touched by participating in a preconception arrangement that was meant to produce a child.

In addition, Guichon (forthcoming) makes the point that it is inappropriate to call the agreements contracts, since the term "contract" implies enforceability. Enforceability of these agreements remains a hotly debated issue in some jurisdictions,[14] and has been explicitly ruled out in others.[15] Consequently, I have changed my terminology with respect to this term as well.

UNCOVERING THE SUBSTRATUM OF A HIDDEN STRATUM

We started this project with the assumption that, besides the agency people, the following people would be involved: the commissioned woman, her husband, where applicable, her children, where applicable, the commissioning man and his wife. In addition, other people, such as other children and parents of any of the participating parties are, of course, important, but we did not expect (and in fact, did not find) any information about them.

This description of the relevant actors assumes a one-to-one correspondence between a commissioned woman, a commissioning man and his wife. This turned out to be false. A commissioning man enters into an agreement with an agency that agrees to find a woman willing to try to bear a child for the man. A successful conclusion involves matching a woman who is willing to serve as a commissioned mother, a man, a successful artificial insemination, a pregnancy maintained to term, the birth of a child, and the surrender of this child from the woman to the man.[16]

However, there is no guarantee that the process will proceed as described without problems. The artificial insemination may not "take." If it does take, the pregnancy may result in a spontaneous abortion, or the child may be stillborn. Consequently, more than one woman may service the same man. Conversely, the same woman may engage in the process more than once, meaning that one woman services more than one man, and/or services the same man more than once. To capture this phenomenon we used as our unit of analysis the case, rather than individual people. Table One summarizes the cases involving Canadians gleaned from Keane's files.

MISCONCEPTIONS: VOLUME TWO

TABLE ONE

CASES INVOLVING CANADIANS IN KEANE'S AGENCY, 1980-1987[1]

	Attorney-Client Agreement		Agreement Signed With Woman[2]		Baby's Birth		Adoption Hearing	
Case 1	Mar	1980	Mar	1980	Feb	1981	Apr	1985
Case 2	Mar	1981	Aug	1981				
			Feb	1982				
			Apr	1983				
			Sep	1983	Nov	1984	Jan	1985
Case 3	Mar	1981	Mar	1981				
			Oct	1981	Sep	1983	Nov	1983
Case 4	May	1981	Sep	1981	Jun	1982	Jun	1983
Case 5	Mar	1982	Apr	1982	May	1983	Feb	1984
Case 6	Jul	1982	Jan	1983				
			Jun	1984				
			Oct	1984				
			Sep	1986[3]				
			Feb	1987				
			Jul	1988				
Case 7	Dec	1982	Mar	1983	Oct	1984	Jan	1985
Case 8	May	1983	Apr	1984	Feb	1986	Apr	1988
			May	1985				
Case 9	Oct	1983	Jan	1984				
			Apr	1985				
			Mar	1985				
			Jul	1986	May	1987	Jul	1987
Case 10[4]	Oct	1983	Jul	1988				
Case 11	N/A		May	1984[5]	Feb	1987	May	1987
Case 12	Nov	1984	May	1985[3]				
			Jul	1986				
			Jun	1987				
			Jun	1988				
Case 13	Apr	1985	May	1985				
			Dec	1985	Sep	1986	Dec	1986

1 For two cases, no data are available.

CASES INVOLVING CANADIANS IN KEANE'S AGENCY, 1980-1987[1]

	Attorney-Client Agreement		Agreement Signed With Woman[2]		Baby's Birth		Adoption Hearing	
Case 14	Jun	1985	May	1986				
			Jan	1987				
Case 15	Dec	1985	Sep	1986				
			Jun	1987				
			Dec	1987				
Case 16	Mar	1986	Feb	1986	Dec	1986	Jun	1987
Case 17	Apr	1986	May	1987	Apr	1987	Jun	1987
Case 18[6]	May	1986	May	1986				
Case 19	May	1986	May	1986	Feb	1987	Apr	1987
Case 20	Sept	1986	Never Selected					
Case 21	Nov	1986	Feb	1987				
			Oct	1987				
Case 22	Mar	1987	Oct	1987				
			Jun	1988				
Case 23	May	1987	Dec	1987				
			Jul	1988				
Case 24	May	1987	Jun	1987[3]				
			Jan	1988				
			Jun	1988				
Case 25	Jul	1987	Aug	1987	May	1988	Jul	1988
Case 26	Jul	1987	Sep	1987	May	1988	Jul	1988
Case 27	Aug	1987	Oct	1987				
			Feb	1988				
Case 28	Aug	1987	Sep	1987	Jun	1988	Aug	1988
Case 29	Sep	1987	Nov	1987	due Aug. 88			
Case 30	Dec	1987	Mar	1988	due Mar. 88			

2 If there are several dates under this heading it means that more than one woman tried to provide a child for the couple. In each case, a new pre-conception contract was signed.

3 indicates that the commissioned woman became pregnant but that the pregnancy ended in a miscarriage. Note: not all miscarriages may be identified.

4 In process of artificial insemination to start a second child for the couple.

5 indicate that the commissioned woman had two miscarriages prior to the birth of the child.

6 In process to start a second child for the couple.

Table 1 demonstrates the wide variety in cases and the impossibility of considering them all to be similar. In terms of length of time, the shortest time interval from when the commissioning man and the agency signed the attorney-client agreement and the adoption of a baby is just less than a year (case 19). Contrast this with case 6, in which a man signed his agreement with the agency in July 1982 and six years later was still trying for a child, in the meantime having utilized the reproductive services of six women.

Popular attention tends to be on the first type of case, in which one woman services one man, and produces a child quickly. We tend to not think about those commissioned women who have miscarriages, sometimes more than once, and who may, in fact, never produce a child for the commissioning man. By contrast, some of the commissioned women may produce more than one child.

In 14 of 30 cases (47 percent) more than one woman serviced one man. In all, the 30 cases listed employed 55 commissioned women, compared to 28[17] commissioning men. Table 2 identifies the cases by number of commissioned women involved.

TABLE TWO

NUMBER OF COMMISSIONED WOMEN INVOLVED PER CASE BY STATUS OF FILE

	Zero	One	Two	Three	Four	Six*
Closed File Successful Pregnancy	0	8	3	0	2	0
Closed File Miscarriage	0	0	1	0	0	0
Closed File No Pregnancy	2	0	1	1	0	0
Open File Pregnancy	0	5	0	0	0	0
Open File No Pregnancy	0	2	3	1	1	1
Total Number of Cases	2	15	8	2	3	1

* There was no instance in which 5 women were employed

Table 2 makes it obvious that the chances a woman will be in a "non-successful" relationship are relatively high, since those cases in which a problem occurs utilize more women. Looking just at the last two columns of table 2, we find three cases in which four women each serviced one man, and one case in which six different women serviced one man!

In the cases available to us, the majority of the commissioned women were married, as were all but one of the commissioning men.

TABLE THREE

MARITAL STATUS OF COMMISSIONED WOMEN AND COMMISSIONING MEN

	Commissioned Women	Commissioning Men
Married	19	26
Single, Separated or Divorced	6	1
No Information	3	5
Total	28	32

It is interesting to note that there is one unmarried man. Although clearly the exception, it is important to realize that these commercial agencies do have the potential to serve as suppliers of children to men who are either not able or not willing to find a woman who wishes to have (a) child(ren) with them in the context of a heterosexual relationship.[18]

ARE PRECONCEPTION AGREEMENTS OPPRESSIVE TO WOMEN?

Sherwin argues in this volume that we must judge the ethical acceptance of a phenomenon within the existing patterns of oppression in our society. She submits that gender and class are two contexts within which we need to place preconception agreements. The data allow us to examine some aspects of patterns of social inequality with respect to the people involved in the transaction.

One common assumption concerning these agreements is that the commissioned women are from a lower class than the commissioning men. This is borne out by our data. Looking first at education, we find that as a group the commissioned women have significantly lower levels of education than do the commissioning men and their wives.

EDUCATION LEVELS ATTAINED BY COMMISSIONED WOMEN
AND COMMISSIONING MEN AND THEIR WIVES*

	Commissioned Women	Commissioning Men	Commissioning Men's Wives
Less than grade 12	2	0	1
Completed Grade 12	13	2	2
Some post-secondary	5	0	1
Completed college and/or university	4	11	10
Completed graduate school	0	4	5**

* Information on four cases is missing   ** Includes Ph.D.s

Clearly, taking education as an indicator, commissioning men and their wives belong to a higher social class than do commissioned women. This is comparable to the situation documented for the U.S. agencies in general (Charo, 1988). With respect to the occupations of the commissioned women, their husbands, where applicable, and the commissioning men and their wives, the results are similar. The commissioned women are either housewives or belong predominantly to the so-called pink ghetto: 10 are housewives, 2 are unemployed, 2 are students, 3 are sales clerks (2 full-time, 1 part-time), and the rest are located (one each) in the following occupations: accounts receivable collector, cashier, co-owner of a tree service, credit administrator, hostess at a restaurant, inventory clerk, nurse, secretary, social work, and waitress.

The husbands of the commissioned women were predominantly blue collar workers: their job categories were (one each) assembly worker in a factory, bricklayer, carpenter, co-owner of a tree-service, electrician, industrial engineer, labourer, machine operator, machinist, mechanic, mechanical engineer, recreation department, sales manager, screen painter, sign painter, student and theatre manager.

Presumably, then, money was a, or *the* major reason for agreeing to become a commissioned woman. Hilary Hanifin, a psychologist at the Center for Surrogate Parenting in California states that nobody in the support group for "surrogate moms" at her center "believes surrogates are doing it just for the money."[19] By contrast, Melia Josephson, a woman who worked as a gestational mother for this center, states:

> The surrogates that I met at the center, in group therapy, a lot of them were doing it for the money. Basically, they went around the room, and said, why are you doing it? Why are you being a surrogate mother? There were answers from: new cars, down payments on house, put themselves through school, help their husband out who wasn't bringing enough home. There was a lot of surrogates doing it strictly for the money.[20]

The commissioning men and their wives belong mostly to the professional class. Their occupations, presented on a couple-by-couple basis, are listed in table 5:

TABLE FIVE
COMMISSIONING MEN'S AND THEIR WIVE'S OCCUPATIONS

Commissioning Man	Commissioning Man's Wife
Bricklayer	Unknown
Business Owner	Business Manager
Carpenter	Supervisor
Construction Business Owner	Nurse
Dentist	Housewife
Doctor-Internist	Doctor-Surgeon
Doctor	Dietician
Engineer	Professor
Engineer	Teacher
Engineer	Secretary
Engineer	Quality Control Manager
Rancher	Teacher
Financial Analyst	Teacher
Lawyer	Bank Worker
Lawyer	Medical Technician
Optometrist	Post Graduate Work
Robotics	Housewife
Self-employed	Teacher
Self-employed	Clerk
Sounds System Designer	Business Manager
Statistician	Teacher
Teacher	Teacher

As a group, then, it is obvious that the commissioning men and their wives would have more money at their disposal than the commissioned women and their husbands. While this is in no way surprising, it is useful to have some empirical confirmation of this fact.

Another relevant factor is age. Supposedly people who are about 40 to 60 will have more financial and other resources at their disposal than will younger people (20 to 30). We did, in fact, find that the age discrepancy between commissioned women and the commissioning men and their wives was significant.

The oldest commissioned women (3 of them) were 33 years of age and the youngest was 19! Their average age was 26.7 years. By contrast, the oldest commissioning man was 59 and the youngest 35, with the average age for commissioning men being 42.9 years. The oldest wife was 56 and the youngest was 34, with an average age of 41 years. In other words, the youngest commissioning man and the youngest wife were older than the oldest commissioned woman. Of the commissioned women, 11 or 46 percent were 25 years of age or younger.

The age of the participants is, of course, consequential to any children that may be born. One wonders what the childhood experience (if, indeed, a child results from the agreement) of some will be. In the case of three commissioning couples, both spouses were over 50 years of age (couple 1: man 59, woman 52; couple 2: man 54, woman 52; couple 3: man 54, woman 56). By the time the children reach age 21, both their parents would be in their 70s or even 80s.

The available evidence suggests that both in terms of class and gender the commissioned women are in an inferior socio-economic situation compared to the commissioning men. Once more, this is comparable to the overall situation in U.S. agencies (Charo, 1988). Given this fact, we can certainly not call the practice a liberating one, but one that reenforces existing patterns of inequality.

This statement is based on statistical data only. It becomes important to the degree it affects the practice of agencies and the manner in which they treat the commissioned women. Two examples of this concern the economic aspects of preconception agreements and the conditions for behaviour laid down by the agencies with respect to the commissioned women.

THE ECONOMICS OF PRECONCEPTION AGREEMENTS

The New York Department of Health has estimated that $33 million have been paid by commissioning couples to agencies in New York (Charo, 1992). Approximately 40 percent of all preconception agreements are estimated to have taken place in New York. (ibid). If this is correct, this is approximately a $82.5 million business. Of the monies expended, about $1 of every $4 actually goes to the commissioned woman (Charo, 1988: 97) — presuming she actually gives birth and relinquishes the child, of course — while the rest goes to various other intermediaries: commercial brokers, attorneys, physicians, psychiatrists, etc.

The fee received by commissioned women upon the surrender of a baby was in 1988 generally $10,000 and is now described as ranging from $10,000 to (in exceptional cases) $20,000 (Charo, 1992). Taking the 1988 figure of $10,000, this amounts to an hourly wage of approximately $1.52 for the woman, counting only the pregnancy and delivery time. This figure ignores the time, effort and discomfort involved in the time preceding a successful pregnancy — which may be considerable, see table 1. The reproductive work of women obviously comes cheap.[21]

REGULATIONS CONCERNING THE COMMISSIONED WOMAN DURING THE AGREEMENT PERIOD

Preconception agreements

typically prohibit the mother from smoking, drinking alcohol, and taking illegal drugs. She must also agree to abide by physician's orders, which may oblige her to undergo amniocentesis, electronic fetal monitoring, or a Cesarean section. Two-thirds of the agency contracts allow the client some control over whether the surrogate mother will undergo chorionic villi sampling, amniocentesis, or abortion, as well as the type of prenatal care she will receive (Charo, 1988: 97).

These are the bare bones of the contracts. However, as Bill Handel, of the Center for Surrogate Parenting explained, the implications of these agreements in regulating and restricting the life of the commissioned woman are much more far-reaching:

The California courts recognize that... the surrogates have no right to the child at all, and six months into the pregnancy a California court issues an order saying the biological parents, no matter where they live, are in fact the legal parents of the child, and the surrogate is a babysitter, albeit a babysitter with a child in utero. And the legal ramifications are fascinating. Does that mean that she can't, for example, take a vacation without informing the parents? That's exactly what it means. She'd be kidnapping their baby if she didn't tell them where she was taking their child.[22]

Given that there is already a strong impetus to involve the judiciary in the surveillance of pregnant women — usually pregnant women of a lower socio-economic status (Bessner in this volume) — the fact that preconception agreements spell out explicit rules of behaviour for pregnant and delivering women is certainly worrisome. First and foremost, the degree of regulation is problematic for the commissioned women. In addition, it may have a spill-over effect for all pregnant and delivering women by reenforcing the tendency to relegate the pregnant woman to the status of a "fetal container" for the baby, or to treat her as, at best, one of two patients: the fetus and the woman. Such conceptualization of pregnancy provides the grounds on which to justify surveillance by others, and the regulation of the pregnant woman's behaviour in order to insure the fetus' safety from the potentially destructive behaviour of its mother. Rather a far cry from providing good prenatal care *to women!*

The sheer existence of a contractual agreement is itself formative of how people understand their own behaviour. "Passivity is valued as good contract-socialized behavior; activity is caged in retrospective hypotheses about states of mind at the magic moment of contracting." (Williams, 1991:43) The odds, then, against "developing a non-exploitative, non-oppressive contractual pregnancy arrangement" (Sherwin in this volume) are, indeed, overwhelming.

CONCLUSION

In a strange way, preconception agreements expose some of the internal contradictions that plague the entire field of reproductive and genetic engineering and put some of the highly problematic aspects into sharp relief.

To begin with, they symbolize the commercialization of childbearing. Preconception agreements may not be the biggest money maker in the human reproduction business, but they are clearly a business (in the commercial version of preconception agreements). More important, and despite the many protagonists who deny that preconception agreements deal with the selling of children (e.g. Andrews, 1988, Dickens, 1988), arguing that only services — the gestation of the child — are sold, the agreements always involve a clause about the possession of children, politely termed adoption. The fact that a child is born within a preconception agreement does not suffice — the child must be surrendered, against a fee, to the commissioning party for the transaction to be completed. This is simply a more obvious and visible manifestation of looking at people as products, rather than as ends in themselves.

As Paul Lauritzen (1990: 43) has noted in a moving personal account of his own experience of infertility, one of the unavoidable consequences of all NRTs is that they treat persons as products.

> *Not only do men and women get treated as products, so do children. The logic here is clear enough. If women are paying for embryos or are being paid for eggs, the embryos and eggs cannot but be understood as products. Because they are products, buyers will place demands on them. We will expect our products to meet certain standards and, if they fail, we will want to be compensated or to return the damaged goods. In a society that sells embryos and eggs for profit, children will inevitably be treated as property to be bought and sold, and just as inevitably it follows that different children will carry different price tags...*

Not all preconception agreements are commercial, however. Another version are so-called "altruistic" preconception agreements, in which a woman carries a child for another woman, often a close relative. This often creates bizarre new family relations, as in the case of the Wesolowski family. Mrs. Wesolowski, a post-menopausal woman of 53, was implanted with the embryo of her daughter-in-law and son. She gave birth to a child who, by one type of reckoning, is her son, by another type, her grandson (Gruson, 1993).

While some suggest that such arrangements constitute the "gift" of a child from one woman to the other (e.g. Laborie, 1988), other authors (e.g. Anleu, 1992, Rowland, 1992) have argued forcefully that they may be as exploitative as commercial ones. A commissioned woman in such an agreement may have as little — or even less — control over her body or her choice to keep the child as a woman who is employed by a commercial agency. Strong support for this argument comes from evidence that commissioned women have unmet needs for affiliation (MacPhee and Forest, 1990) that make them particularly vulnerable to promises of close relationships with the commissioning couple. This would make women highly vulnerable to family pressures.

When the commissioned woman is a close family member, such as a sister, mother, mother-in-law, the very factors which make this arrangement appealing also pose special dangers should the relationship sour. A recent Shirley Show[23] dealt with the issue of "Sisters who have babies for sisters." One pair of sisters appeared together and sang the praises of this arrangement. It was clear that the sisters maintained a close and emotionally supportive relationship with each other.

In the other case, a commissioned woman and her teenage daughter were present, while the commissioning woman was not. The commissioned woman, and her daughter from her marriage, were extremely distressed and unhappy because they had lost not only a child/sibling, but also any meaningful contact with the sister/aunt. The grandmother of the child in question, mother to both sisters, supported the commissioning woman.[24] The commissioned woman, as a consequence of an act that she had hoped would strengthen family ties, thus found herself without access to her genetic and gestational child, separated from her sister and mother and with severely strained relations with the remaining family members. Her daughter and her other children have effectively lost a sibling, an aunt and uncle, access to a cousin (there was already a child in the other family), and a grandmother. The suffering was palpable.

Most importantly, preconception agreements expose, in their non-commercial as well as commercial variants, the profound double standard with respect to the importance of genetic relatedness that characterizes the debate surrounding NRTs.

At first, this presents itself as a sexual double standard. A famous and often-quoted passage by Judge Sorkow in the Baby M. trial (the judgment was later overturned by a higher court), argues that the father "cannot purchase what is already his," although the mother can clearly sell what is hers. However, upon closer reflection it becomes obvious that the double standard operates between commissioning and commissioned person. In the case of preconception agreements the two double standards coincide.

Looking at the new reproductive technologies in general, we find that the genetic relation between parent and child is variously upheld as the single most important factor, or considered of no importance. The factor that determines whether it is of overriding or of no importance is the status of the gamete donor/recipient as either commissioning or commissioned person, and it applies to both women and men.

Consider the case of artificial insemination by donor. It is primarily used on married women. The woman's husband, who has no genetic relationship to the ensuing child, becomes the legal father. The sperm donor is legally and socially declared a non-father, although genetically he is the father of the child. Where legislation concerning filiation in the case of AI exists, that is what is being stipulated. In this instance, the recipient woman is the commissioning party, and her genetic relationship to the child is of undoubted importance. Her husband acquires parenthood via his marriage to her, and the sperm donor (vendor) is the commissioned party for whom genetic relatedness to the child is deemed irrelevant.

In the case of preconception arrangements, the roles shift. In this instance, the sperm donor (otherwise legally considered a non-father) becomes the undoubted father due to his genetic relatedness to the child. He also happens to be the commissioning party. His wife acquires parenthood via marriage to him and adoption of the child, and the birth mother is the commissioned party for whom genetic relatedness to the child is assumed to be irrelevant.

We found that in 50 percent of the commissioning couples[25] there were already one or more children in the family. Unfortunately, the data do not allow us determine whether these were biological children of both spouses, or only of one. One child was identified as adopted. Given the ages of the commissioning couples, as well as various individual cases that have been reported (e.g. Radovsky, 1993), it seems reasonable to speculate that in most instances these would have been children that the wife brought into the marriage. If such was the case, it would suggest that his genes suffice to make a child a child of the marriage, but hers don't.

Matters get even more complicated when we are dealing with what is sometimes called "full," "total" or "gestational surrogacy." This occurs when a woman gives birth, within the context of a preconception agreement, to a child that is genetically the child of the commissioning woman and her partner. These services are now offered by agencies specializing in commercial preconception agreements. We are then dealing with a commissioning couple and a gestational mother.

So far, in law, the mother was always the woman who gave birth. The precept that "The mother is always known" (mater semper certa est) is premised on this assumption. The first case which tested this notion was the recent case of Anna Johnson. She gave birth, within the context of a preconception agreement, to a baby to whom she is not genetically related, and subsequently sued for access to the child. She lost her case because "she and the child are genetic hereditary strangers" (Annas, 1991: 36; see also Brahams, 1991) There may have been a racist element informing this judgement — Anna Johnson is black (see Pollit, 1990) and she happens to be the commissioned party. The Court of Appeal also affirmed that the egg donor was the "real" mother (Capron, 1991).

Contrast this with the situation of egg donation, now practiced in a number of programs in Canada, as well as world-wide. In these cases, the egg recipients, who are the commissioning women, are without doubt seen to be the mother of the ensuing child, while the genetic relatedness of the egg donors to the children is seen as irrelevant and they are regarded as nonmothers. They are also the commissioned women.

The evidence suggests then, that the importance of the genetic relatedness between parent and child is a flexible matter that is either promoted as being the most important factor or totally irrelevant to establish parenthood. It depends on whether a potential parent is the commissioning or commissioned party. These facts can be summarized as follows in table 6:

TABLE SIX

		Do genetics predict who counts as parent?	Does commission status predict who counts as parent?
AI by Donor	Sperm donor	No	Yes
	Recipient's husband	No	Yes
AI in preconception arrangements	Sperm donor	Yes	Yes
	Commissioned mother's husband	Yes	Yes
	Commissioned mother	No	Yes
	Sperm donor's wife	No	Yes
Egg donation in clinic program	Egg donor	No	Yes
	Egg recipient	No	Yes
Egg donation in pre-conception arrangement	Egg donor	Yes	Yes
	Egg recipient	Yes	Yes

So do genetics determine parental status? It depends on whether you are commissioned or commissioning.[26] If you are the commissioning party, your sperm or eggs — if they were used — establish parentage beyond any doubt. If they were not used, the person whose egg, uterus or sperm was used was only a "substitute" and her or his genetic relationship to the child is only of interest if it will help produce a "gloriously healthy, plump and squalling newborn."[27] Genetic relations, after all, seem to be endowed with or stripped of importance to service other interests.

Once we cease to think of the commissioned women as disembodied "uteri" and see them as women — in economic straits, and with families of their own — it becomes apparent that preconception arrangements for the production of children pose a danger not only to the commissioned women and their potential offspring, but to our entire way of dealing with motherhood.

NOTES

1 From the Presidential Address of the 55th annual meeting of the Pacific Coast Obstetrical and Gynecological Society, Sandberg, 1988, p. 1442.
2 All quotes in this paragraph are from Sandberg, 1989.
3 I would like to thank Ann Webb for conducting these searches for me.
4 Rowland (1992) has performed a useful service by pulling together a lot of these individual cases. However, the selection of the cases generated in this manner remains problematic.
5 The empirical data are drawn from Eichler and Poole, 1988.
6 This counts Keane's two agencies of the time as one.
7 This was due to a stroke of good luck. In May 1987, I found myself on a popular panel discussing the

ethics of surrogacy with a number of other people, including Noel Keane. After the public discussion was over, I asked Noel Keane wether he would allow a student access to his files, should I ever find one who wanted to write a thesis on the topic of surrogacy. He said he would be willing to allow access. I never found such a student, but in 1988, when the Law Reform Commission of Canada asked me to conduct the study, I called Noel Keane up, reminding him of our conversation and the promise he made then. I found a student, Phebe Poole, who was able to travel to Michigan. She looked at the information contained in the files, we devised a way in which to extract this information, and she subsequently gleaned the available information from all files in Keane's office involving Canadians, with the names and other identifying information blanked out.

8   We used two estimates in our study. There was some uncertainty how many cases there were in Quebec. The low estimate, therefore, is 104 cases, the high estimate 118. That is the figure I have cited here. See Eichler and Poole, 1988, for further details on this matter.

9   Sandberg, p. 1446.

10   See below.

11   Although not specifically stated, the context makes it clear that this refers only to babies born through the arrangements of commercial agencies.

12   There were 7 cases in which Keane's agency used a Canadian as a commissioned woman, but of these, only one is included in the analysis, since she served as a commissioned mother for a Canadian couple. On the other six commissioned women, unfortunately no information was available to us. This brings the total number of cases involving Canadians through Keane's agency to 38, although we shall only be analyzing 32 of them.

13   See Eichler, 1988.

14   The Ontario Law Reform Commission (1985) argued strongly for making surrogacy contracts enforceable, while the Quebec Council on the Status of Women (1988) argued equally strongly that they should be unenforceable. Quebec has since passed a law to that effect.

15   In the U.S., 18 states have either banned or restricted commercial surrogacy: Arkansas, Arizona, Florida, Indiana, Kentucky, Louisiana, Michigan, Nebraska, Nevada, New Hampshire, New Jersey, North Dakota, Oklahoma, Oregon, Utah, Virginia, and Washington. In addition, New York passed a law in 1992 outlawing payment to a broker and making any agreement without legal standing in a court. This law will go into effect in July 1993 (Charo, 1992).

16   Other agencies offer other forms of "gestational surrogacy," including egg donation, and carrying a couple's fetus to term through IVF.

17   The number is 28 rather than 30, since in 2 cases no contract with a woman was signed; see table 2. Please keep in mind that the number of total cases varies slightly from table to table, due to missing information in some of the files.

18   The Office of Technology Assessment reported only nine single men as clients of all commercial surrogacy agencies, and the number of homosexual individuals or couples are consistently reported as no more than 1 percent, see US (1988: 69).

19   From the script of the NFB/CBC/Cinefort film by Gwynne Basen "On The Eighth Day: Perfecting Mother Nature. Part I: Making Babies."

20   Ibid., with slight grammatical corrections.

21 See also Anderson, 1990.

22 From the script of the NFB/CBC/Cinefort film by Gwynne Basen. This involved a case of what is called by some "total surrogacy" — the child was genetically the child of the commissioning couple. The child has been reduced to the status of a thing that is simply placed into a uterus, while the commissioned woman is reduced to the status of a carrier who is treated as if she was in bondage to the commissioning couple (or the agency, as the case may be).

23 Aired January 1993.

24 Personal conversation. I participated as an "expert" on the show. Of course, the only experts were the people who had experienced the consequences of such an arrangement.

25 This is a higher proportion than reported for all U.S. agencies, in which the figure is reported to be 25 percent (Charo, 1988).

26 A report on the Swedish approach to NRTs states simply : "Surrogate motherhood is contrary to the basic principles of Swedish law, according to which the woman who gives birth to a child is its mother. If anyone proposes to take charge of the child the only way is adoption, which is not allowed on the basis of a surrogacy contract. The committee found no reason for any changes in the provisions." (Sverne, 1990: 468) What a simple and elegant solution!

27 Sandberg, p. 1446.

REFERENCES

Anderson, ELizabeth S. "Is Women's Labor a Commodity?", *Philosophy and Public Affairs*, 1990, Vol. 19, #1, pp. 71-92.

Andrews, Lori B. "Surrogate Motherhood: The Challenge for Feminists," in *Law, Medicine and Health Care*, 1988, Vol. 16, #1-2, spring-summer, pp. 72-80.

Anleu, Sharon Roach. Surrogacy: For Love But Not for Money?," *Gender and Society*, 1992, Vol. 6, No. 1, pp. 30-48.

Annas, George J. "Crazy Making: Embryos and Gestational Mothers," *Hastings Center Report*, Jan.-Feb. 1991, Vol. 21, No.1, pp. 35-38.

Brahams, Diana. "Medicine and the Law," *The Lancet*, Jan. 1991, Vol. 337, pp. 228-229.

Capron, Alexander Morgan. "Whose Child Is This?," *Hastings Center Report*, Nov.-Dec. 1991, Vol. 21, No. 6, pp. 37-38.

Charo, R. Alta. "Legislative Approaches to Surrogate Motherhood," *Law, Medicine and Health Care*, 1988, vol. 16, 1-2, spring-summer, pp. 96-112.

Charo, R. Alta. "USA: New York Surrogacy Law," *The Lancet*, 1992, Vol. 340: August 8, p. 361.

Chesler, Phyllis. "Pound of Flesh," *New Statesman and Society*, March 9, 1990, Vol. 3, No. 91, pp. 29-31.

Dickens, Bernard. "Conference", in *Sortir la maternité du laboratoire*. (Actes du forum international sur les nouvelles technologies de la reproduction, organisé par le Conseil du statut de la femme.) Gouvernement de Québec, Conseil du status de la femme, 1988, pp. 178-186.

Eichler, Margrit. "Preconception Contracts for the Production of Children — What are the Proper Legal Responses?", in *Sortir la maternité du laboratoire*. (Actes du forum international sur les nouvelles technologies de la reproduction, organisé par le Conseil du statut de la femme.) Gouvernement de Québec, Conseil du status de la femme, 1988, 187-294.

Eichler, Margrit and Phebe Poole. *The Incidence of Preconception Contracts for the Production of Children among Canadians*. A Report Prepared for the Law Reform Commission of Canada. [Montreal:] 1988.

Gruson, Lindsey. "When 'Mom' and 'Grandma' Are One and the Same," *New York Times*, Feb. 16, 1993, pp. B1 and B5.

Guichon, Juliet. "An Analysis of the Common Perception of the Practise of Preconception Arrangements and an Analysis of the Proponents' Arguments, The Choice of Two Models and a Legislative Proposal," unpublished manuscript.

Laborie, France. "La radicalité de meres porteuses," in *Sortir la maternité du laboratoire*. (Actes du forum international sur les nouvelles technologies de la reproduction, organisé par le Conseil du statut de la femme.) Gouvernement de Québec, Conseil du status de la femme, 1988, 205-214.

Lauritzen, Paul. "What Price Parenthood?," *Hastings Center Report*, March/April 1990, Vol. 20, #2, pp. 38-46.

MacPhee, David and Kathy Forest. "Surrogacy: Programme Comparisons and Policy Implications," *International Journal of Law and the Family*, 1990, Vol. 4, pp. 308-317.

Ontario Law Reform Commission. *Report on Human Artificial Reproduction and Related Matters*. [Toronto:] Ministry of the Attorney General, 1985.

Québec. Ministère de la santé et des services sociaux. *Rapport du comité de travail sur les nouvelles technologies de reproduction humaine*. Quebec: 1988.

Radovsky, Vicky Jo. "Deidre Hall: My hands and heart are full," *First for Women*, May 17, 1993, Vol. 5, #20, pp. 36-38.

Rowland, Robyn. "The depersonalisation of birth mothers: so-called 'surrogacy'", in *Living Laboratories: Women and Reproductive Technologies*. Bloomington: Indiana University Press, 1992, pp. 156-198.

Sverne, Tor. "Bio-technological developments and the law," *International Social Science Journal*, 1990, Vol. 42, No. 4, pp. 465-473.

Vandelac, Louise. "La 'media-éthique' des technologies de reproduction," Paper given at the Coloque éthique et communication, Cerisy-La-Salle, June 1992.

United States of America Congress. Office of Technology Assessment. *Infertility. Medical and Social Choices*. Washington, D.C.: Government Printing Office, 1988.

Williams, Patricia J. "Reflections on Law, Contracts, and the Value of Life," *Ms.* May/June 1991, Vol. 1, No. 6, pp. 42-46.

PART VI

PUBLIC POLICIES

Several groups and organizations have taken public stances on the new reproductive and genetic technologies. The positions of the National Action Committee on the Status of Women (Canada), the Council for Responsible Genetics (U.S.A.) and the Feminist International Network of Resistance to Reproductive and Genetic Engineering (international) are reprinted on the pages that follow.

A

THE NATIONAL ACTION COMMITTEE ON THE STATUS OF WOMEN

The National Action Committee on the Status of Women (NAC) is the largest feminist organization in Canada. Since its inception in 1972, NAC has been at the heart of the struggle for women's equality in Canada. At present, NAC includes about 500 member groups reflecting the diversity of Canadian women and their communities.

NAC has played a leading role in publicly opposing the proliferation of the reproductive and genetic technologies in Canada and in condemning the failed process of the Royal Commission. Resolutions have been voted on and approved at three NAC annual general meetings and a series of recommendations were included in the organization's brief presented to the Royal Commission on The New Reproductive Technologies.

1. IN VITRO FERTILIZATION

For the last fifteen years, IVF has been marketed to the public as a "medical miracle." The real miracle is that a set of experimental procedures — which have never been properly evaluated or subjected to controlled research trials, that have an 85% failure rate and present serious health risks to women and children — should even be called a medical "treatment."

The emphasis on the technological "cure" has diverted both attention and resources away from research into the real causes and prevention of infertility. In 1990, the Canadian Government spent $3.5 million on research in reproductive technology and $400,000 on public health research into the causes of infertility.

Infertility is created in a society that ignores the public health issues of safe work places, better programs to deal with sexually transmitted diseases, improved measures to reconcile workplace and family responsibilities, and the need to clean up the environment. Instead, we deal with infertility solely as an individual problem requiring individual and very expensive high-tech experimentation.

There are tremendous economic interests pushing the expansion of these technologies. One example is the drug company Serono Canada. It is part of the transnational drug company, the Ares-Serono Group, and the biggest producer of drugs used for ovulation stimulation. In 1991, the company sold $625 million dollars worth of drugs world-wide.

Serono owns and operates IVF clinics in England, including Bourn Hall, where Robert Edwards, the IVF doctor who has been called the "laboratory father" of the first "test-tube baby," continues his work. As well, individual doctors and hospitals benefit from the money and the prestige associated with these reproductive technologies.

The women who undergo IVF are subjected to known and suspected health risks from the "fertility" drugs used to increase the production of eggs. If a woman does conceive through IVF, the pregnancy will be more problematic and medicalized.

It is not just women who are affected by these technologies. Babies born as part of a multiple birth are more likely to be premature and of low birth-weight, and to suffer from the health problems associated with those conditions.

Rather than spend huge sums on experimental procedures that will assist a tiny minority of women, governments should be devoting resources to the prevention of infertility and to social programmes that truly support women and children.

RESOLUTION:

Be it resolved that NAC call on federal and provincial governments to halt further expansion of IVF facilities and place existing facilities under rigorous scrutiny along the lines suggested by the World Health Organization in 1990.

Be it further resolved that NAC demand significant resources be devoted to infertility prevention campaigns which can be combined with existing prevention issues such as AIDS and STD prevention, workplace health and safety, and patient information.

2. EMBRYO RESEARCH

Human embryo research is a controversial undertaking. In Canada, it is nevertheless proceeding unimpeded because all levels of government have sat on their hands, allowing uncontrolled proliferation as they waited for the report of The Royal Commission on the New Reproductive Technologies.

The techniques that enable the laboratory creation of human embryos are expanding rapidly. The use of ova stimulation drugs in combination with *in vitro* fertilization and embryo freezing techniques have produced a new category of potential human life, the "surplus" embryo. The ability to mature human eggs in the lab has made female cadavers and even fetuses a source of research embryos.

The technology is also available to biopsy and screen human embryos. The procedure is called preimplantation diagnosis of the embryo. It has been banned in Germany but here in Canada the first program that would use this technique has been set up at The University Hospital in London, Ontario in collaboration with the IVF clinic there. This marks a great departure from the original use of IVF as a treatment for infertility.

The embryo manipulation techniques used in pre-implantation diagnosis are very similar to the ones now being used to split and clone human embryos. This technology, like most other of the reproductive technologies, comes from the animal breeding industry. It is part of a continuum that is transforming human procreation into an industrial process.

From the screening of embryos it is only a small technical step, though a huge social one — to the modification of the human embryo through germ-line genetic manipulation. In such interventions, all future generations of the modified organism are affected by the genetic changes made. It is here that we pass beyond human reproduction and move into conscious human fabrication.

Without human eggs there are no embryos, and women are (for now) the only source of eggs. But the mainstream debate on this issue has been concerned only with the status of the embryo itself. Questions are posed about whether and when it is a human being. There are debates about ownership and management. NAC insists that the experimentation on women's bodies that results in the creation of research embryos become a central element in the ethical examination of embryo research.

NAC has always fought for women to have control over their reproductive lives. NAC believes that these technological developments, left unchallenged, will result in the removal of women from the process of human reproduction.

Given the global scope of the research and applications, NAC also believes that only internationally co-ordinated multi-government action can slow down, re-direct, and in some cases stop, the proliferation of this enterprise.

RESOLUTION:

Be it resolved that NAC oppose the creation of human embryos for research purposes and call for a ban on embryo-manufacturing technologies, including ova maturation, artificial-uterus research and cloning.

Be it further resolved that NAC oppose any commercialization of embryos.

Be it further resolved that NAC call for a ban on pre-implantation diagnosis of the human embryo and call on the Government of Canada and the Government of Ontario to ensure that this procedure will not be performed and to represent this as Canada's position internationally.

Be it further resolved that NAC call for a ban at all levels of Government, both federal and provincial, on the funding of embryo research.

Be it further resolved that NAC call on the Government of Canada to include initiatives that proactively pursue the tenets of domestic policy at the international level, via the United Nations and other international bodies and agreements.

Be it further resolved that NAC call for a ban on germ-line genetic manipulation of the human embryo.

3. SEX SELECTION

At present, prenatal determination of fetal sex is possible via chorionic villus sampling (CVS), amniocentesis and ultrasound. Pre-pregnancy techniques include preimplantation diagnosis of the embryo and sperm selection. Today, sex selection is a commercial enterprise in Canada. Clinics, operating as money-making ventures, sell their services to parents wishing to increase their chances of having a child of the selected sex.

The practice of sex selection, in the context of patriarchal social relations, is virtually always used to eliminate female embryos or fetuses. NAC finds this practice misogynist and abhorrent.

NAC is particularly alarmed and appalled by the position the Society of Obstetricians and Gynaecologists of Canada (SOGC) has taken on this issue. The SOGC has adopted a recommendation in which they are prepared to consider sex selection for the purpose of "family completion" (their term). This utterly retrograde notion of the "complete" family reinforces sex/gender stereotypes and turns children into commodities, valued not for who they are but for being of the "right" gender.

"Family completion" bears no relationship to issues of health or wellness. NAC considers the SOGC position to be an unethical abuse of medicine and technology and demands it be withdrawn.

RESOLUTION:

Be it resolved that NAC call on governments to prohibit the licensing of clinics specializing in sex selection.

4. PRECONCEPTION AGREEMENTS ("SURROGACY")

Commercial contract motherhood represents an extension of the exploitation of women and the ascendancy of property and contract law over the rights of the gestating mother. In this way, the interests of affluent men and women are validated over those of poor women, often women of colour. It also accelerates the process of the commodification of both children and women's reproductive capacities.

RESOLUTION:

Be it resolved that NAC call on governments to ban commercial contract motherhood and, until such legislation is created and enforced, all commercial motherhood contracts be made legally unenforceable.

5. PRENATAL DIAGNOSIS

NAC is committed to protecting women's reproductive rights. The increasing "biologization" or "geneticization" of ill-health and lack of "fitness" acts as an ideological and practical barrier to addressing the economic and social factors which are in fact responsible for the vast majority of such problems. The prevalence of babies with low birth weight — most commonly related to the mother's socio-economic status and the conditions of her life before, during and after pregnancy — is far greater than the prevalence of Down syndrome or neural tube defects. Yet, expensive screening programs are becoming routine practice while early prenatal nutritional support is still not available. Men's violence against pregnant women is also ignored.

NAC is concerned by the proliferation of prenatal testing and the subsequent pressures put on individual women to become the agents for "quality-control" in human procreation.

Prenatal testing such as amniocentesis, chorionic villus sampling and alphafetoprotein screening are the most widely used and "normalized" of all the new reproductive and genetic technologies. Ultrasound is now used in almost 90% of pregnancies in Canada.

These technologies validate a ranking of worthiness of human life and, despite the options they may open for individual women, they contain and encourage a eugenic dynamic in society.

RESOLUTION:

Be it resolved that NAC call for the directing of public resources to address conditions of maternal well-being through programs for maternal and community health (physical and emotional) in relation to the importance of these factors in causing infant disability.

Be it further resolved that NAC call for a collective, social and economic analysis of ill-health and disability and reject the individualized, genetic formulation that has become the dominant model.

Be it further resolved that NAC work towards stopping the momentum of prenatal screening becoming a routine part of prenatal care.

Be it further resolved that NAC call for an independent (consumer- and academic-led, rather than medical-led) study whose purpose is to generate broad public debate on the impact of prenatal diagnosis in the context of women's lives; in particular, examining and making recommendations on the following:

1) The economic and political dynamics of testing.

2) The prevalence and nature of iatrogenic (physician caused) infant disability.

3) The incidence of men's violence during pregnancy and the effect of this brutalization on women and newborns.

6. GENETIC TESTING

The number and range of genetic tests available has expanded greatly over the past few years. Unless strict guidelines and mechanisms of control are set in place, proliferation will make genetic tests acceptable as the basis for decision-making about individuals by predicting their "future" health; by identifying their genetic "predisposition" to medical conditions such as cancer, cardiovascular diseases and mental disorders. While the reliability of these tests in forecasting the future health of individuals is questionable, the prevention and cure of these medical conditions is taking second place to the advances made in genetic testing.

In a world where reproductive and genetic technologies are committed to the creation of "perfect" human beings, genetic testing serves to increase forms of discrimination.

RESOLUTION:

Be it resolved that NAC demand that genetic testing not become a part of routine health services.

Be it further resolved that NAC oppose genetic discrimination and call for legal and social measures prohibiting discrimination in education, employment, insurance, housing and other areas, based on present or predicted medical status or hereditary traits.

Be it further resolved that NAC support absolute and legally binding guarantees of confidentiality to protect information obtained from genetic screening. The information should not be released to anyone without the informed consent of the screened person or her/his legal guardian.

Be it further resolved that NAC call for advocate, non-biased counselling to every individual offered genetic testing, to inform them of the option to refuse tests and of the benefits and risks of doing so. The Government of Canada should ensure that refusal to undergo testing will not lead to discriminatory practices.

7. THE ROYAL COMMISSION ON THE NEW REPRODUCTIVE AND GENETIC TECHNOLOGIES

In November 1993, the Royal Commission on the New Reproductive Technologies presented their final report and 293 recommendations. NAC considers the Royal Commission to have been a deeply flawed process. There was no genuine public consultation. Neither was there the much needed public education process that NAC had demanded in their brief to the Commission.

No modern society can call itself a meaningful democracy if it cannot control the direction of science and industry. But informed democratic decision making depends on having access to the kind of thoughtful, critical, in-depth information that Canadians have not had access to.

Those progressive groups who have very serious concerns about the development and regulation of these technologies must have the opportunity to evaluate the report and recommendations and to consult with other like-minded organizations. Intervenor funding from the government is crucial at this time to permit that process to take place.

RESOLUTION:

Be it resolved that NAC lobby the federal, provincial and territorial governments for funds, specifically 1% of the 29.5 million dollar budget of the Royal Commission on the New Reproductive and Genetic Technologies, thereby permitting NAC to initiate and coordinate a regional, national and international process of active, meaningful and genuine education, discussion, and debate regarding the new reproductive and genetic technologies and the consequential impact on all women and children, in particular lesbians, women with disabilities, women of colour and society in general.

Be it further resolved that NAC work with the federal government to demand the release and full disclosure of all research commissioned by the Royal Commission on the New Reproductive Technologies.

The final report and recommendations of the Royal Commission are alarming. The serious eugenic implications of these technologies are never addressed. Among the other things missing is an analysis of the economic interests that drive the development and expansion of these technologies.

NAC is extremely concerned about the proposed regulatory body. The Regulatory Commission would have enormous power and authority with no accountability, while at the same time offer limited possibility for genuine public participation. The proposed composition of the regulatory body, based on representation by individuals, excludes the involvement of organizations concerned about the development and use of these technologies.

NAC is very concerned that given the structure and composition of the proposed regulatory body, experimentation on women, children and procreation will be legitimized and institutionalized. We have seen how it is harder to discontinue a practice after it has been put in place. It is for this reason that NAC is calling for a moratorium, until democratically determined regulatory agencies are put in place.

RESOLUTION:

Be it resolved that NAC demand that the federal, provincial and territorial governments immediately impose a moratorium on the following:

• the opening of any new IVF clinics

• the introduction into clinical practice of any new reproductive technology or genetic technology included in the mandate of the Royal Commission on the New Reproductive Technologies.

• the expansion of existing technologies until such time as democratically determined regulatory agencies have been put in place.

Be it further resolved that NAC ensure that the Medical Research Council of Canada and any other funding agency, including those controlled by private industry, impose a moratorium on the funding of any research projects aimed at expanding clinical applications of reproductive and genetic technologies included in the mandate of the Royal Commission on the New Reproductive Technologies. This moratorium must exist until and during a genuinely democratic process of discussion and debate determines the nature of the necessary regulatory agencies.

B

THE COUNCIL FOR RESPONSIBLE GENETICS

The Council for Responsible Genetics (CRG) is a U.S. based non-governmental organization of scientists and non-scientists. The CRG has been one of the leading organizations worldwide to consistently challenge the direction of biotechnology.

The mission of the CRG is:

- to promote public discussion about new genetic technologies
- to alert the public to the social and environmental problems arising from these technologies
- to bring these technologies under public control
- to support developments in biotechnology in the public interest

The central principles that guide the vision of the CRG are:

- the public must have access to clear and understandable information on technological innovations
- the public must be able to participate in public and private decision-making concerning technological developments and their implementation
- new technologies must meet social needs
- problems rooted in poverty, racism and other forms of inequality cannot be remedied by technology alone.

Abridged versions of two policy positions developed by the CRG are presented here.

Biologists and physicians as well as social theorists and politicians have tried to understand how physical and social traits are passed on to successive generations. This interest in heredity has had a range of motivations and effects:

(1) Conservative and progressive thinkers alike have often labored under the mistaken assumption that our environment can be molded, but that our biology is unchangeable, and have therefore tried to identify fixed quanta of biological inheritance and to sort them from social and other environmental influences.

(2) As scientists have devised methods to study the components of organisms at the molecular level, their focus has shifted from explanations at the level of organisms to chromosomes, genes, DNA molecules, and the nucleotide bases that give DNA its specificity.

(3) Molecular geneticists assume that a better understanding of these smaller components will provide better insights into how whole organisms function, individually and in society. However, this reductionist view ignores the fact that molecules and sub-cellular structures, cells and tissues, and organisms and, indeed, societies all interact with each other and with everything that goes on around them, so that it is impossible to predict how changes in the molecules or genes will affect what happens at other levels.

At present, molecular biologists in the United States, Europe, and Japan[2] have begun to tackle the enormous project of identifying and mapping the fifty to one hundred thousand genes on the twenty-three pairs of human chromosomes and of sequencing the approximately three billion pairs of nucleotide bases of which these genes are composed. The international project, which goes under the name HUGO (for Human Genome Organization), was initiated by some thirty-two scientists from the participating countries. The U.S. project, known as the Human Genome Initiative, was begun at the instigation of the Department of Energy, but now has its headquarters at the National Institutes of Health and is under the direction of Francis Collins. The Department of Agriculture and the National Science

Foundation plan to participate as well. The fiscal year 1995 budget for the NIH's part of the project is $153 million.

PROMISES:

The project promises to improve scientific knowledge about how both genes and organisms function. At the practical level, it promises to improve the ability to predict, diagnose, and cure genetic disease. The pharmaceutical industry is interested in developing molecular probes for specific genetic lesions, which could be used to diagnose "defects" in fetuses, children, or adults. It is hoped that therapies could be developed once it is possible to locate and isolate the genes involved in specific disease. For example, once a gene known to mediate a particular disease has been isolated, it might be relatively easy to identify its gene product(s) and use them to cure or ameliorate the disease. Alternatively, it might be possible to administer the gene in some form of gene therapy.

CRITIQUE:

A. Scientific:

The underlying assumption that motivates most genome research is the scientifically inaccurate belief that genes represent a "blueprint" for an organism and "control" the way the organism develops and functions. In this reductionist view, humans are "readouts" of our genes, whose sequence and composition conceal a gold mine of information about our biology and behavior. Obviously, genes are important components of an organism that make significant contributions to its metabolism. But they are not autonomous. Their structures and functions are affected by what goes on around them.

The office of the Human Genome Initiative will no doubt sponsor research that will advance the understanding of genetics and therefore of genetic components of health and disease. However, knowing the sequence of an organism's genes will not make it possible to predict how that organism will function because genes are not "blueprints" of the organism. They are merely one of many important elements that participate in its metabolism and development. Genes specify the amino acid sequence of proteins, which in this context are often referred to as "gene products." But each gene product (hence each gene) can affect many traits of an organism; conversely, many gene products (hence many genes) usually contribute to each trait. For example, when the gene that specifies the structure of human growth hormone (a protein) was transferred into the DNA of a mouse embryo, the animal grew to twice its normal size. However, when the same gene was transferred into a hog embryo, the animal's size did not change, but it was leaner than normal. In other words, the way the gene functioned depended on what was going on in the rest of the organism.

Moreover, in humans the same gene clearly can exert different effects in different individuals. For example, molecular biologists know how the gene for sickle cell hemoglobin differs from that for normal hemoglobin. For about thirty years they also have known the precise molecular difference between these two types of hemoglobin. Yet that has not made it possible to predict, or understand, why some people who have sickle cell anemia are seriously ill from earliest childhood, while others do not show symptoms till much later in life, and some of them only quite mild ones. Nor has any of this knowledge helped produce effective therapies, much less cures. Similarly, a few people with Huntington disease, a gene-based progressive, degenerative disease of the nervous system, have experienced the first symptoms in childhood, while the majority experience them in their middle years, and a few not until old age. This is why it is erroneous to believe that knowing the sequence and composition of all the genes on the human chromosomes — a gigantic task — will tell us a very much about ourselves or even help cure many diseases.

Advocates of the Human Genome Initiative point to the fact that it will provide tools for the early diagnosis of gene-based diseases. They also claim that this will speed the discovery of cures. But early diagnosis is of questionable value in the absence of therapies, and specifying the genetic basis of a disease will only rarely produce better therapies in the foreseeable future.

For the reasons we have discussed, information at the level of the gene cannot be readily translated into useful information at the level of cells, tissues, or whole organisms. Traditionally, scientists have deduced the presence of genes, as well as their functions, by looking at the way organisms differ from one another. It is not at all obvious that that scenario can be usefully played backwards, that is, that one will be able to identify a gene's critical function, or functions, once one has identified, located, and isolated it.

The main point is that even if we knew everything we could about the human genome, we would know only a tiny piece of the story. The most that the complete sequence of an organism's genes can tell us is what proteins that organism can make. Such a list of ingredients cannot tell us how they will interact and operate together. Anyone who has tried to prepare more than the simplest dish from a recipe knows that having a complete list of ingredients, including the sequence in which to add them, does not guarantee the outcome.

B. Economic:

At present, scientists, physicians, venture capitalists, and industrialists are involved with gene mapping and with genetic diagnosis and gene-based therapy. In their search for funding, they often describe genes as though they were all-important and determined who we are and what we do. This draws attention away from other biological processes as well as from the many societal factors that enter into the picture. Genes have their part to play in the ways people function, but they are always only part of the story. At a time of increasing conservatism and shrinking budgets for measures which could ameliorate the various problems that confront our society — from the growth of an impoverished, drug and alcohol addicted portion of our population to our increasingly health-imperiling working and living environments — focusing on genes as the cause of our various problems will make it more difficult to enact appropriate social policies. Yet, scientists and the media at present sound a steady drumroll of publicity claiming that genes are being identified that confer "tendencies" to develop the range of addictions and diseases that plague us.

There is also the question to what extent this project will draw funds away from other potentially interesting and productive areas of biology. Its proponents argue that by turning biology into "big science" and linking it more inextricably with industry and government, the project will, in fact, bring more money into biology than would happen otherwise. They say that without that kind of money, it would be difficult, if not impossible, to develop the kinds of tools necessary to understand how genes operate. In all likelihood it would simply take longer. Since all that money is going into looking for genes and analyzing them, and since they are only one component of the total picture, the genome project vastly exaggerates the importance of genes — especially at this time, when a deteriorating environment and economy make it increasingly difficult for most people to live healthful lives.

C. Discrimination:

Individuals experience discrimination whenever they are judged not for who they are or what they can do, but on the basis of their membership in a particular group, defined by skin color, sex, or some other characteristic. In addition, genetic discrimination may involve predictions about the future. Yet genetic predictions entail a considerable degree of uncertainty about the extent to which the trait in question will be expressed or whether it will be expressed at all. If the genetic trait confers evident disabilities, a person may be protected by civil rights laws that prohibit discrimination for reasons of disability. However, if someone shows no signs of disability, but a genetic diagnosis suggests that she or he may become disabled at some undetermined future date, that person may not be protected by current civil laws.

The Human Genome Initiative is bound to lead to improved techniques for various forms of genetic diagnosis and DNA-based identification for a range of diseases and disabilities that could not be predicted before. As procedures are simplified and used more widely, the opportunities for genetically-based discrimination will increase. This is most likely to become apparent in the areas of employment and insurance and in forensics. DNA-based, compulsory identification of specific groups (e.g., all those convicted of a sex offense or other violent crime) or individuals raises numerous unresolved ethical and political questions. Finger printing and social security numbers entered our society to facilitate identification in specific, limited contexts. They are now used widely and individuals have little, if any, recourse to refuse without drawing suspicion upon themselves. The same can be expected to happen with DNA-based identification, which potentially contains more information and therefore poses considerably greater risks to privacy and civil liberties.

D. Other Social Policy and Ethical Issues:

Concepts of health and normalcy: The renewed emphasis on genes as "causes" of a wide range of health and social problems raises a host of ethical issues. First and foremost is that while some diseases and disabilities are clearly disabling, and the people who have them, and their families, urgently wish for improved diagnostic techniques and for therapies that can ameliorate or cure them, many inherited disorders are minor or can be readily relieved. Most of us have one or more of them. Health and disease, normality and abnormality are culturally constructed categories on which there is no general agreement. In particular, the criteria scientists and physicians use often are not the same as those used by other segments of society. This raises the question, what will be defined as a "genetic lesion" and who among us will be defined as "abnormal." We have no proper medical or social definitions of "normal," since the term signifies a distribution around a mean. And there is no general agreement as to where "normal" shades into "abnormal."

In the absence of valid social mechanisms for setting up appropriate categories, there are obvious dangers to labelling various inherited characteristics as diseases or disabilities. Once wide-spread, socially stigmatized behaviors, such as alcoholism or other forms of addiction become included under the umbrella of "genetic diseases," increasing amounts of economic and social resources will go into finding biomedical "cures" while social measures will be discredited and short-changed. The history of eugenics in the United States and Europe gives reason for concern. The eugenics movement included alcoholism, along with pauperism and various forms of mental illness and "deficiency," among the inherited traits for which compulsory sterilization was socially and medically approved as a "cure."

The focus on genes, and the effort to discover genetic components or tendencies for all sorts of diseases that have obvious environmental components, is problematic not only because it draws attention away from the political changes needed to deal with them in other ways. These very political changes would also be required to render genetic and medical information useful. Economic barriers prevent large numbers of people from taking advantage of medical information that is already on hand. This is likely to get worse for gene-based medical information because it will necessarily be expensive to obtain and act on.

Prenatal diagnosis: A number of ethical issues are implicit in the use of prenatal diagnosis for inherited disorders. There are the problems of definition and labelling. There is also the obvious problem that, while many disabilities have a range of severities, prenatal tests give only yes or no answers, so that prospective parents are forced to make difficult procreative decisions in the face of limited, sometimes questionable, information. And at present, the only recourse offered to most people whose tests reveal that their future child will have a disability is abortion.

In the present climate of increasingly restricted access to abortion, especially for poor women, the decision to abort in the context of prenatal diagnosis is likely to be hemmed in in one of two ways, both of them bad. One is that diagnoses of inherited disabilities will be granted the status of exceptions in laws restricting access to abortion, thus increasing the stigma on people with inborn disabilities as well as the pressure to abort fetuses that manifest them. The other is that they will not be exempted, so that only affluent women will have access to prenatal diagnosis and abortion, by going to states in which these are available.

Privacy rights: Many ethical issues surround the disclosure of genetic information. What rights does an individual have not to disclose such information to present or prospective employers, insurers, or spouses, and to other family members? If someone who has a genetic disease decides to keep that fact secret, to which, if any, of these people should a health care provider be permitted, or indeed mandated, to disclose the information? These are some of the many thorny issues our society has not confronted and almost surely is not ready to deal with equitably. Yet the Human Genome Initiative will provide a host of such data, whether we are ready for them or not.

The NIH program has decided to allocate between one and five percent of its budget to research into ethical consequences of the Genome Initiative. Such research projects at best can yield worthy suggestions, with no assurance that they will be implemented. Yet it is certain that employers, insurers, and others who stand to gain financially or politically from obtaining genetic information about other people will make every attempt to gain access to it once it exists. It is irresponsible to acquire and store such data before confidentiality can be assured.

NOTES

1 This is an abridged version of the original CRG document. A full report can be obtained directly from the CRG at 5 Upland Road, Suite 3, Cambridge, MA, 02140. (617) 868-6870

2 And now Canada, too (eds).

POSITION PAPER ON HUMAN GERM LINE MANIPULATION

PRESENTED BY COUNCIL FOR RESPONSIBLE GENETICS HUMAN GENETICS COMMITTEE FALL, 1992

The Council for Responsible Genetics (CRG) strongly opposes the use of germ-line gene modification in humans. This position is based on scientific, ethical, and social concerns.

WHAT IS "GERM-LINE MANIPULATION?"

The undifferentiated cells of an early embryo develop into either germ cells or somatic cells. Germ cells, or reproductive cells, are those that develop into the egg or sperm of a developing organism and transmit all its heritable characteristics. Somatic cells, or body cells, refer to all other cells of the body. While both types of cells contain chromosomes, only the chromosomes of germ cells are passed onto future generations.

Techniques are now available to change chromosomes of animal cells by inserting new segments of DNA into them. If this insertion is performed on specialized or differentiated body tissues, such as liver, muscle, or blood cells, it is referred to as somatic cell gene modification, and the changes do not go beyond the individual organism. If it is performed on sperm or eggs before fertilization, or on the undifferentiated cells of an early embryo, it is called germ cell or germ-line gene modification, and the changes are not limited to the individual organism. For when DNA is incorporated into an embryo's germ cells, or undifferentiated cells that give rise to germ cells, the introduced gene or genes will be passed on to future generations and may become a permanent part of the gene pool.

Deliberate gene alterations in humans are often referred to as "gene therapy." The Council for Responsible Genetics (CRG) prefers to use the terms "gene modification" and "gene manipulation" because the word "therapy" promises health benefits and it is not yet clear that gene manipulations are beneficial.

WHAT IS THE FEASIBILITY OF MODIFYING THE GERM-LINE OF HUMANS?

Both somatic and germ-line modification are widely performed on laboratory animals for research purposes. Somatic gene modifications have already been performed on humans and additional experimental protocols are being approved by the National Institutes of Health in increasing numbers.

No published reports have yet appeared on germ-line modification in humans, but there appear to be no technical obstacles to such experiments, and articles proposing these procedures are becoming more and more common in the literature (1,2,3). Germ line gene modification has actually proved technically easier than somatic modification in mice and other vertebrate animals which have been employed as "models" for human biology in the past because the cells of early embryos incorporate foreign DNA and synthesize corresponding functional proteins more readily than most differentiated somatic cells. A widely-reported example of the successful experimental use of the germ-line technique was the introduction of an extra gene that specified growth hormone into fertilized mouse eggs. In the presence of the high levels of growth hormone produced, the mice grew to double their normal size. Germ line techniques are also being used in attempts to modify farm animals, with stated goals of increasing yields or enhancing nutritional quality of meat and other animal products.

Given what has been accomplished in animals, the only remaining technical requirements for germ-line gene modification in humans are procedures for collecting a woman's eggs, fertilizing them outside her body, and implanting them in the uterus of the same or another woman, where they can be brought to term. These are already well established procedures for humans and are widely used in *in vitro* fertilization clinics.

WHAT ARE THE TECHNICAL PITFALLS?

Current methods for germ-line gene modification of mammals are inefficient, requiring the microinjection of numerous eggs with foreign DNA before an egg is successfully modified. Moreover, introduction of a foreign gene (even if there is a copy of one already present) into an inappropriate location in an embryo's chromosomes can have unexpected consequences. For example, the offspring of a mouse that received an extra copy of the normally present *myc* gene developed cancer at 40 times the rate of the unmodified strain of mice (4).

Techniques to introduce foreign DNA into eggs, however, are constantly being improved and eventually will be portrayed as efficient and reliable enough for human applications. It may soon be possible to place a gene into a specified location on a chromosome while simultaneously removing the unwanted gene. This will increase the accuracy of the procedures, but does not eliminate the possibility that gene combinations will be created that will be harmful to the modified embryo and its descendants in future generations. Such inadvertent damage could be caused by technical error, or more importantly, by biologists' inability to predict how genes or their products interact with one another and with the organism's environment to give rise to biological traits. It would have been impossible to predict, *a priori*, for example, that someone who has even one copy of the gene for a blood protein known as hemoglobin-S would be protected against malaria, whereas a person who has two copies of this gene would have sickle cell disease.

This unpredictability applies with equal force to genetic modifications introduced to "correct" presumed disorders and to those introduced to enhance characteristics. Inserting new segments of DNA into the germ-line could have major, unpredictable consequences for both the individual and the future of the species that include the introduction of susceptibilities to cancer and other diseases into the human gene pool.

WHAT ARE THE SOCIAL AND ETHICAL IMPLICATIONS OF GERM-LINE MODIFICATION?

Clinical trials in humans to treat Adenosine Deaminase Deficiency — a life threatening immune disorder — and terminal cancer with somatic gene modification are already in progress and experiments to treat diabetes and hypertension are under development. It is important to distinguish the ethical problems raised by these protocols from the additional, and more profound questions raised by germ-line modification. While the biological effects of somatic manipulations reside entirely in the individual in which they are attempted, such treatments are not strictly analogous to other therapies with individual risk. Radiation, chemical or drug treatment can be withdrawn if they prove harmful to the patient, while some forms of somatic modification cannot. Thus, somatic gene modification requires a person to forfeit his/her rights to withdraw from a research study because the intervention cannot be stopped, whether harmful or not. Valid objections have also been raised to the fact that the first somatic gene modification experiments, involving Adenosine Deaminase Deficiency, were carried out on young children who were not themselves in a position to give informed consent. While it appears that somatic gene modification techniques will be used increasingly in the future, the CRG urges that they be used with greatest caution, and only for clearly life-threatening conditions.

Germ line modification, in contrast, has not yet been attempted in humans. The Council for Responsible Genetics opposes it unconditionally. Ethical arguments against germ-line modification include many of those that pertain to somatic cell modification, as well as the following:

• Germ line modification is not needed in order to save the lives or alleviate suffering of existing people. Its target population are "future people" who have not yet even been conceived.

• The cultural impact of treating humans as biologically perfectible artifacts would be entirely negative. People who fall short of some technically achievable ideal would increasingly be seen as "damaged goods." And it is clear that the standards for what is genetically desirable will be those of the society's economically and politically dominant groups. This will only reinforce prejudices and discrimination in a society where they are already prevalent.

• Accountability to individuals of future generations who are harmed or stigmatized by wrongful or unsuccessful germ-line modifications of their ancestors is unlikely.

In conclusion, the Council calls for a ban on germ-line modification.

REFERENCES

1. Walters, Leroy, "Human Gene Therapy: Ethics and Public Policy," *Human Gene Therapy*, v.2, pgs. 115-122, 1991.
2. Working Group on Genetic Screening and Testing, Report of Discussions in Genetics, Ethics and Human Values, XXIVth CIOMS Conference, Tokyo and Inuyama, Japan, 24-26 July 1990.
3. Buster, John E. and Carson, Sandra A., "Genetic Diagnosis of the Preimplantation Embryo," *American Journal of Medical Genetics*, v. 34, pp. 211-216, 1989.
4. Leder, A. et al, "Consequences of Widespread Deregulation of the c-myc Gene in Transgenic Mice: Multiple Neoplasms and Normal Development," *Cell*, v. 42, p. 485, 1986.

NOTE

1 For a full copy of this document, write directly to the CRG at 5 Upland Road, Suite 3, Cambridge, MA, 02140. (617) 868-0870

C

1. We, the women from Australia, Austria, Bangladesh, Brazil, Canada, Denmark, Egypt, Fiji, France, Federal Republic of Germany, Hong-Kong, Holland, India, Indonesia, Japan, Malaysia, Mauritius, Norway, Pakistan, Peru, Philippines, Sri Lanka, South Korea, Spain, Sweden, Switzerland, U.K., Uganda, U.S.A., Zambia have met in Comilla, Bangladesh, to share our concern about reproductive and genetic engineering and women's reproductive health. We feel an urgent need to halt the political decisions which are leading to the rapid development and increasing application of these technologies.

2. Initial experiences with reproductive and genetic engineering all over the world show that these technologies are aggravating the deteriorating position of women in society and intensifying the existing differences among people in terms of race, class, caste, sex, and religion. These technologies also contribute to the further destabilizing of the already critical ecological situation.

3. Genetic and reproductive engineering are part of an ideology of eugenics which we oppose. In this ideology human beings are viewed as inherently inferior or superior. This leads to degradation, discrimination and elimination of oppressed groups; be they women, disabled, people of certain colors, races, religions, class, or caste. Similarly, traits of animals and plants are arbitrarily valued as being desirable or undesirable and become subject to genetic manipulation.

4. Eugenics justifies the political strategy used by those in power to divide and rule.

5. Women from the participating countries described how eugenic ideology and racism are the basis of population control policies. We resist population control policies and methods. They hide the true roots of poverty as exploitation

by the rich. They reduce women to their reproductive organs. We object to women being used as experimental subjects by science, industry, and government.

6. Genetic and reproductive engineering, as well as population control, are introduced and promoted on the grounds that they solve problems such as hunger, disease and pollution. In reality, however, they divert attention from the real causes and are incapable of solving these problems. Nor do they reflect women's demands and needs.

7. Genetic and reproductive engineering claim to offer unlimited control over all life forms, but tinkering with genetic codes opens up a truly uncontrollable situation of "runaway designer genes" and unintended consequences. These changes will be particularly hazardous because a chain reaction will be set in motion which cannot be traced back to its origins. The effects produced cannot be countered. They will be irreversible.

8. In our increasingly materialistic and consumer oriented world, genetic engineering is promising unlimited diversity. But to live in a man-made patriarchal world where everything has been tampered with will be to live with the ultimate limitation. Our present finite world of resources offers a richer diversity than that promised by genetic engineering with its selective, eugenic, and patriarchal philosophy.

9. Genetic and reproductive engineering are a product of the development of science which started off by viewing the whole world as a machine. Just as a machine can be broken down into its components, analyzed and put back, living beings are seen as consisting of components which can be viewed in isolation. Aspects of nature which cannot be measured or quantified are seen as subjective and of no value and are therefore neglected. In their ignorance or disregard of the complex interrelationships in life, scientists collaborate with industry and big capital and believe they have finally acquired the power to create and reconstruct plants, animals, other forms of life and, possibly soon, even human beings. We oppose this patriarchal, industrial, commercial and racist domination over life.

10. In our work of bearing and raising children, caring for the sick or disabled, growing, preserving, and preparing food, materials for clothes and other basic human needs, we women have developed and passed on for generations a

wealth of knowledge and skills about dealing with all of nature in a compassionate, humane, and ecologically sustainable way. We realize that this knowledge and these skills, as well as the contributions of women to the arts, crafts, culture, and social relations are generally not recognized as having value in mainstream science, philosophy, or technology. But these have been and still are vital for the survival of human beings and all of nature. They are valuable human achievements and resources. We want to renew, reaffirm and build upon this female tradition.

11. We strongly believe that reproductive and genetic engineering cannot meet the needs of women or enhance their status in today's societies. We therefore demand the participation and recognition of women in all spheres of life. We want women to have access to resources, income, employment, social security, and a safe environment at work and at home. Quite fundamentally, we demand living and working conditions that assure a life of human dignity for all women worldwide.

12. We demand access for girls to practical knowledge, resources, and skills that are in women's best interest and further women's well being. These include an education about taking care of primary health needs including nutrition. This will empower women and increase women's general health, reduce morbidity and mortality of women and children. Such primary health care will reduce the number of children born with mental and physical disabilities and also reduce infertility.

13. We demand knowledge and access to safe contraception which does not harm women's bodies. We reject any coercion, be it through force, incentives, or disincentives in the name of population control policies, such as enforced sterilization particularly in camps and in target oriented policies. We demand a stop to the use of dangerous IUDs, unsafe injectables, hormonal implants, such as Norplant, and other hormonal contraceptives as well as anti-fertility vaccines.

14. We support the recovery by women of knowledge, skill, and power that gives childbirth, fertility and all women's health care back into the hands of women. We demand recognition, support and facilitation of the work of midwives and reestablishment of midwifery services under the control of women.

15. We demand literature be distributed and education be given about adverse effects of all contraceptive methods.

16. We demand contraceptives for men be developed and that also men be made responsible for contraception.

17. We demand the United Nations and the governments of the respective countries stop population control policies as preconditions for developmental aid.

18. We support the exclusive rights of all women to decide whether or not to bear children without coercion from any man, medical practitioner, government or religion. We demand that women shall not be criminalized for choosing and performing abortion.

19. We oppose the medicalization and commercialization of the desire of women for motherhood.

20. Internationally, we demand that conditions be created under which social parenthood in a variety of forms meets the needs of children and people who wish to care for children. In particular maternity and child care should be a social concern rather than the responsibility of individual women.

21. We condemn men and their institutions that inflict infertility on women by violence, forced sterilization, medical maltreatment and industrial pollution, and repeat the damage through violent "repair" technologies.

22. Given the continuing deterioration of women's lives through the application of patriarchal science and technology, we call for an international public trial on medical crimes against women to be organized by women.

23. We demand research into the prevention of infertility as well as an end to the stigmatization of the infertile. Infertility needs to be acknowledged as a social condition and not as a disease.

24. We protest the use of *in vitro* fertilization in countries that wish to increase or decrease births. It is a dangerous dehumanizing technology. It uses women as living test sites and producers of eggs and embryos as raw material to enable scientists to work towards further control over the production and quality control of human beings and international business to accumulate profit. Furthermore, it is a failed technology which also takes away resources from basic reproductive health needs.

25. The social discrimination against women is aggravated through the technologies of sex determination and sex preselection resulting in a growing

adverse sex ratio in some countries. We demand a ban on such applications of these technologies.

26. We are against any kind of bias and discrimination against disabled people including that of genetic screening and counselling. We particularly oppose the Human Genome Project within this context. Prenatal diagnosis, genetic screening, and genetic counselling do not offer the solution for disability. Instead we demand the elimination of hazardous drugs, radiation, hazardous chemicals at the workplace and in the environment and a solution to the problems of malnutrition and preventable infectious diseases.

27. Disabled people must be integrated into society and accorded full respect as human beings. The responsibility for caring for the disabled must be of social rather than of individual concern.

28. We condemn any national and international traffic in women, eggs and embryos, human organs, body parts, cells, or DNA (genetic substance) especially for purposes of reproductive prostitution which exploit women as human incubators, in particular poor women and women in poor countries. We also strongly protest against the existence of "baby farms" and commercial adoption and surrogacy agencies.

29. We oppose the deliberate release of genetically manipulated organisms worldwide because of its unpredictable and irreversible effects on our environment and health. We also consider the use of genetic engineering in laboratories and factories (biotechnology) to be tantamount to deliberate release, because genetically manipulated organisms can be released accidentally.

30. Deliberate release of genetically manipulated organisms and safety standards in factories and research institutions are of international concern and cannot be decided by certain governments only. The impossibility of democratic control of genetic engineering on a national and international level leads us to reject all forms of genetic engineering.

31. We strictly reject any laws which allow patenting of life forms and processes utilizing life forms.

32. We condemn the use of poor countries as test-sites for genetically

engineering organisms or other products of genetic engineering such as the bovine growth hormone, rabies vaccine, etc.

33. We fear that the development and application of gene technology in agriculture will repeat and aggravate the damage done by the green revolution; in particular that it will increase the economic dependency of poor countries on rich countries and concentrate power in the hands of a few, both nationally and internationally.

34. We demand an end to technologies and policies which result in natural food being converted into more expensive unnatural food.

35. We oppose the criminalization and repression of women who are critical of genetic engineering and reproductive technologies or who are against the dehumanizing technologies.

36. We want appropriate technologies that do not violate human dignity and relations. We want them to be reversible, that is to be error friendly, and contribute to preserving biological, cultural, and social diversity of all living beings. The technologies must be suited to collective decision-making and democratic participation and control.

37. We women gathered here are natural and social scientists, doctors, lawyers, health activists, journalists, demographers, development workers, community organizers, teachers, social workers, academics, who have been actively involved in issues related to women, health, human rights, education, responsible science, technology, and agriculture with a women-oriented perspective in both professional and political work. Having shared our experiences, insights and knowledge, we reaffirm our deep commitment to continue and intensify our work towards a humane and just world for all. We will continue this work, despite the numerous restraints and increasing repression, both political and professional, which we face.

38. We appeal to all women and men to unite globally against dehumanizing technologies and express our solidarity with all those who seek to uphold and preserve the diversity of life on our planet and the integrity and dignity of all women.

25th March 1989 Kotbari, Comilla, Bangladesh

ABOUT THE AUTHORS

Rosanna Baraldi holds master's degrees in psychology and communications. She has taken part in research projects on women's questions and for some years has been working with the group D.E.S. Action Canada. Currently she is completing a doctorate in sociology on the ethical discourse in the fields of human reproductive technologies.

Gwynne Basen is a writer and film maker. She is the director of *On the Eighth Day: Perfecting Mother Nature*, a series of two films on the new reproductive and genetic technologies, co-produced and distributed by The National Film Board of Canada. She also co-produced, *I Lease Wombs, I Don't Sell Babies*, a video tape on the subject of preconception agreements, distributed by Cinéma Libre, Montreal. She is currently co-chair of the Reproductive Technologies Committee of The National Action Committee on The Status of Women (NAC). She lives in Montreal with her husband and two children.

Ronda Bessner, B.A. Honours (McGill) 1977, B.C.L. (McGill) 19481, LL.M. (Harvard) 1986, was called to the Ontario Bar in 1983. She is currently practising Criminal Law and she teaches Children and the Law at the University of Toronto Law School. From 1989-1992, Ms. Bessner was at the Ontario Law Reform Commission. She is the author of several articles and cases comments in the areas of criminal law, evidence, constitutional law and family law.

Karen Capen MA, BCL, LLB is currently completing the Law Society of Upper Canada's bar admission requirements, and is a doctoral candidate with a dissertation topic on human reproduction ethics.

Gena Corea, born in 1946, became an investigative reporter in 1971 and her articles have appeared in such publications as the *New York Times*, *Ms.*, *Commonwealth*, *The Progressive*, *Omni*, and *Mother Jones* and in many anthologies published in the United States, Britain, Germany, France and Australia. She is the author of *The Hidden Malpractice: How American Medicine Mistreats Women* and *The Mother Machine: Reproductive Technologies from Artificial Insemination to the Artificial Womb*. She is the co-founder of the Feminist International Network of Resistance to Reproductive and Genetic Engineering (FINRRAGE), and its journal and she is now associate director of the Institute on Women and Technology.

Lynda Davies has been active in the movement to end violence against women and children for ten years. She has worked with the Assaulted Women's Helpline, the Barbara Schlifer Commemorative Clinic and Education Wife Assault in Toronto and was a founding member of the Canadian Health Alliance to Stop Therapist Exploitation Now (CHASTEN). She currently resides in Ottawa, teaches at the School of Social Work, Carleton University and is a member of Women's Health Interaction, a feminist health collective, and the Women's Alliance for Reproductive Health.

Margrit Eichler is a professor of Sociology at the Ontario Institute for Studies in Education (OISE). She has been following the NRGTs since the first case of a preconception arrangement in Canada in 1982. Her books include *The Double Standard* (1980), *Families in Canada Today* (1988), *Nonsexist Research Methods* (1988).

Kate Fillion is the author of *Lip Service: Challenging the Sexual Script of the Modern Woman*. She is a contributing editor to both *Saturday Night* and *Toronto Life* magazines, and was a columnist for the *Globe and Mail* for three years. She has written for a wide variety of Canadian magazines and newspapers, and won a national magazine award for her article "Fertility Rights, Fertility Wrongs."

Donna Launslager is the mother of five children including eight-year-old quadruplets. She has been a member of the Parents of Multiple Births Association of Canada's Board of Directors for the last five years and is currently Health & Education Director and Project Coordinator for POMBA's Canadian Multiple Birth Needs Assessment Project funded by Health and Welfare Canada's "Brighter Futures" program.

Abby Lippman is based in the Department of Epidemiology and Biostatistics at McGill University and is Chair of the Human Genetics Committee of the Council for Responsible Genetics. Her research focuses on the application of genetics from a feminist perspective, emphasizing the increasing geneticization of health and illness and the biopolitics of biomedicine. She and her two children have lived in Montreal for the past 20 years, but her Brooklyn-accented French immediately reveals her New York City origins.

Maggie MacDonald is currently pursuing a Ph.D. in social anthropology at York University.

Heather Menzies is a writer, mother, lecturer, gardener and activist in the women's movement and peace movement. Her books include: *The Railroad's Not Enough, Canada Now* (1978), *Women and the Chip* (1981), *Computers on the Job* (1982), *Fastforward and Out of Control* (1989) and *By The Labour of Their Hands: The Story of Ontario Cheddar* (1994).

Karen Messing is professor of biology and director of CINBIOSE, (Centre pour l'étude des interactions biologiques entre la santé et l'environment) of the University du Québec à Montréal. She received her Ph.D. in biology in 1975 from McGill University. Her research centres on women's occupational health and she has published papers on the effects of work on human genes and on the menstrual cycle. She is currently studying the workload of hospital cleaners.

Lisa M. Mitchell received her PhD in anthropology from Case Western Reserve University earlier this year. Her principal research areas are in studying science and medicine, particularly obstetrics and reproductive technology. She teaches anthropology part-time at Concordia University in Montréal and is engaged in research on the controversy about the health effects of electromagnetic fields.

Gail Ouellette is a molecular geneticist who has worked on mechanisms of mutagenesis and carcinogenesis. She has a Ph.D in molecular biology and her present interest is the understanding of biological mechanisms underlying occupational health problems, particularly in the fields of reproduction, genotoxicity and cancer.

Susan Sherwin teaches philosophy and women's studies at Dalhousie University. Her principle areas of research interest are in health care ethics and feminist theory. She is the author of *No Longer Patient: Feminist Ethics and Health Care* (Temple University Press, 1992). She is a co-editor of *Health Care*

Ethics in Canada (HBJ Holt, forthcoming) and is Principal Investigator on a 3-year SSHRC Research Network Grant supporting collaborative research to explore feminist perspectives on questions in health care ethics.

Harriet Simand, upon learning that she was a DES daughter, tried to get information about diethylstilbestrol but met with a blank wall. She founded DES Action Canada in 1982 with a grant from Health and Welfare Canada. It is now a nation-wide organization with a doctor's referral list, an extensive reference library, a staff trained to respond to the questions of DES daughters, mothers, and sons, and a newsletter on DES research and related issues. Harriet is currently practising law in Toronto.

Laura Sky is an independent documentary film-maker who focuses on social and political issues in Canada. In the past ten years, she has produced and directed three feature-length documentaries on the ethics, politics and economics of health care in Canada. She is currently the national secretary of the National Action Committee on the Status of Women.

Louise Vandelac has a doctorate in sociology from the University of Paris. She is a professor in the Department of Sociology at l'Université du Québec à Montréal. She was a member of the National Council on Bioethics for Research on Human Subjects from 1988 to 1991 and a Commissioner on The Royal Commission on the New Reproductive Technologies from 1989 to 1991. She has both researched and published widely on the questions of the ethical, economic and social issues that relate to the new reproductive technologies and on the role of the media in this area.

MISCONCEPTIONS: THE SOCIAL CONSTRUCTION OF CHOICE AND
THE NEW REPRODUCTIVE AND GENETIC TECHNOLOGIES
VOLUME 1
is also available. It contains:

Part I: Setting the Context
Part II: Eugenics: From Then To Now
Part III: The Royal Commission on New Reproductive
Technologies

You can order a copy through your bookstore or by calling
Voyageur Publishing at (613) 925-2111 fax: (613) 925-0029
(messages can be left 24 hours per day).

All bookstore orders will receive a trade discount.
You will be billed when the book is shipped.

Voyageur Publishing
considers complete unsolicited manuscripts.
If you have a manuscript please address it to:
Voyageur Publishing/New Manuscripts
Maple Pond, Maple Ave. RR#2 Prescott, Ontario K0E 1T0

PLEASE NOTE:

The Editors of this book have donated their royalties to the
National Action Committee on the Status of Women (NAC).

Both the Publishers and the Editors believe that NAC is doing
essential work with respect to the New Reproductive and Genetic
Technologies and for women in general.

You can contribute to NAC's work. Donations should be made
payable to the NAC Charitable and Educational Trust and are tax
deductible.

You can reach NAC at: 234 Eglinton Ave E. Suite 203, Toronto,
Ontario M4P 1K5   tel: (416) 932-1718

2290